diversion (da - vur' - zhan) n. [ME. *diversioun* < ML. *divusio* (for LL. *deversio*)] 1. a diverting, or turning aside (*from*) [*diversion* of funds from the treasury] 2. distraction of attention [*diversion* of the enemy] 3. anything that diverts or distracts the attention; specif., a pastime or amusement.

Websters New World Dictionary

To my children, for their never ending support, and to Ellen Fahy, for continuing encouragement.
E.S.

To Nancy, who knows why.
LeC.B.

To my husband, Ben Farney, and to LeClair Bissell, for being such truly good friends and extending my limits.
E.W.

Chemical Dependency in Nursing

CHEMICAL DEPENDENCY IN NURSING

THE DEADLY DIVERSION

Eleanor Sullivan, PhD, RN

LeClair Bissell, MD, CAC

Etta Williams, MPA, RN, SCADC

ADDISON-WESLEY PUBLISHING COMPANY
Health Sciences Division, Menlo Park, California
Reading, Massachusetts ▪ Menlo Park, California ▪ New York
Don Mills, Ontario ▪ Wokingham, England ▪ Amsterdam
Bonn ▪ Sydney ▪ Singapore ▪ Tokyo ▪ Madrid ▪ Bogota
Santiago ▪ San Juan

Sponsoring Editor Nancy Evans
Production Supervisor Wendy Earl
Text and Cover Designer Andrew H. Ogus
Cover Photographer Richard Tauber
Manuscript Editor Wendy Earl
Desktop Publisher Robin Ann Gold

The author and publishers have exerted every effort to ensure that drug selection and dosage set forth in this text are in accord with current recommendations and practice at the time of publication. However, in view of ongoing research, changes in government regulations and the constant flow of information relating to drug therapy and drug reactions, the reader is urged to check the package insert for each drug for any change in indications of dosage and for added warnings and precautions. This is particularly important where the recommended agent is a new and/or infrequently employed drug.

Library of Congress Cataloging-in-Publication Data
Sullivan, Eleanor J., 1938-
    Chemical dependency in nursing.

    Bibliography: p.
    Includes index.
    1. Nurses—Substance use. 2. Substance abuse—Treatment.
3. Nursing—Psychological aspects.
I. Bissell, LeClair. II. Williams, Etta. III. Title.
[DNLM: 1. Nurses—psychology. 2. Nursing. 3. Substance Abuse.
4. Substance Dependence. WM 270 S949c]
RC564.5.N87S85 1988   616.86′0088613   87–31887

ISBN 0-201-07581-4

ABCDEFGHIJ–BA–891098

Addison-Wesley Publishing Company
Health Sciences Division
2725 Sand Hill Road
Menlo Park, California 94025

FOREWORD

More than 20 years ago, I worked as a young staff nurse on a general medical unit that was considered a training and testing ground for new graduates. About the only thing that made this floor bearable was its head nurse. She was tall, white-haired, tough, compassionate, competent, and fair. Patients loved her, physicians respected her, and her staff idolized her. I thought surely she was the best nurse in the hospital, probably in the whole world. So, when I first discovered discrepancies in the narcotics records, I was sure there was a reasonable explanation. When her behavior changed, I was sure it was merely fatigue. And when she was stripped of her job, her license, and her freedom, I was devastated. Not *because* of her but *for* her. Although not, surely not, as devastated as she.

Surveys of health professionals indicate that most of us view chemical dependency as a treatable disease *unless* the chemically dependent person is a colleague. Then, we try to act as if such behavior results from a moral defect.

Research also shows—repeatedly—the effect that professionals have on one another. When exposed to excellent practice and compassionate behavior, professionals emulate one another. When exposed to sloppy practice and harsh behavior, unfortunately they also tend to emulate one another. These findings are independent of background, education, and experience. Apparently values—including professional values—are not learned from books and somehow embedded in our characters. Rather they are transmitted by direct contact and require frequent renewal for survival. Apparently we refresh and renew one another's values through demonstrating them, or they wither and die. This reinforcement is necessary with our nursing practice, and it is also true in our collegial relationships.

Nursing exists only in its practice and in its practitioners. Each day in practice you and I create or diminish the profession. *The nurse is nursing* and anything that undermines or destroys the practitioner undermines and destroys the profession.

Unquestionably, chemical dependency undermines and, if untreated, destroys the practitioner and wounds the profession. Estimates of nurses affected by chemical dependency (primarily alcohol and other drugs) range between 10% and 20% of all actively practicing nurses. Easy access, the mistaken belief that professionals can "self-medicate" safely, the "drug culture" in which many of us grew up are just a few of the reasons.

CHEMICAL DEPENDENCY IN NURSING: The Deadly Diversion represents a breakthrough toward ending the "throwaway nurse syndrome." It is the first comprehensive guide on how to deal effectively and humanely with the problem, from identification of the chemically dependent nurse through intervention, treatment, and reentry into the job market.

The authors bring rich and varied experience and knowledge to this topic; all three have worked with chemically dependent nurses and have written and lectured widely on the topic. Their goals in writing this book were, first, to bring the problem out in the open and, second, to provide practical, hands-on help in dealing with it.

They offer no easy answers; instead, they make an eloquent plea for collegial commitment to finding solutions—commitment from *both* management and staff. They ask that all of us care enough to help one another for our own sake and for the sake of the profession.

From a purely practical viewpoint, we can no longer afford to "throw away" between 10% and 20% of existing nurses when we are facing a shortage of up to a quarter of a million nurses by 1992. For the sake of patients, families, and institutions, we cannot afford to ignore the problem. Impaired practice is a very real danger...a deadly diversion of precious human resources.

This new book offers hope and a means to end the "throwaway nurse syndrome."

Leah Curtin, MS, MN, RN, FAAN

Adapted by permission from Editorial Opinion, *Nursing Management*, July, 1987

CONTENTS

Continued

Continued

PREFACE

This book is for people in health care who are concerned about the nurses and their families who suffer from alcoholism or addiction to other drugs. This includes nursing administrators and risk managers, employee assistance program personnel, members of regulatory boards, nursing educators, friends, and colleagues.

We explore the nature and extent of chemical dependency in the nursing profession and the efforts undertaken to confront it, the characteristics of chemically dependent nurses, and the special problems they face as members of their profession. We review the advantages and disadvantages of different approaches and suggest solutions to some of the common problems encountered. We also present current research data and suggest additional work that needs to be done.

We approach this topic with certain basic assumptions. First, chemical dependency is a disease, not a lifestyle or a moral problem; and second, sustained recovery can only be achieved through ongoing, lifelong, and total abstinence from the mood-altering drugs of addiction. A variety of terms are used in conjunction with this disease, and there are numerous interpretations and definitions of addiction. In our context, the term chemical dependency refers to addiction to alcohol and other mood-altering drugs.

We hope our readers are interested in learning about chemical dependency and in applying what they learn. This is not, however, a

game for amateurs; too much is at stake. To become knowledgeable
and effective, you do not have to have a history of personal involvement
with addictive illness. You must, however, examine your own
attitudes about addiction and your preconceptions about nurses and
the health care professions. You must also take a hard look at your own
and your family's patterns of drinking and other drug use. As we
emphasize repeatedly, honesty is essential. Denial of reality is the
major obstacle in coping with the disease of chemical dependency for
both the addict and his or her associates.

In presenting our knowledge and insights about chemical dependency, we have made some assumptions about our readers. We assume that they are concerned and caring and that they are seeking
positive solutions to the problems of chemical dependency—solutions
that can restore the life of the person suffering from the disease, as well
as help and protect the friends, families, co-workers, patients, and
institutions affected by the afflicted person.

As professionals and as employers it is hard to accept this illness
within our ranks. It may be shocking—even horrifying—to learn that
a colleague or employee is chemically dependent. But if we react with
outrage and punishment alone, we convey the message that these matters must stay hidden. As we discuss, covering up and ignoring this
disease has been dangerous and costly. By facing the problem and
providing ways to overcome it successfully, we help individuals in
need *and* we benefit the reputation of our profession and our health
care institutions.

For those readers who are already involved in assisting and treating
chemically dependent nurses, we appreciate your efforts. Nurses can
be difficult patients. We hope this book will help you understand the
special factors that are important to consider when dealing with
chemically dependent nurses.

About the Authors

We have among us the combined experience of personal recovery from alcoholism and other drug addiction, of living with a chemically dependent person, of professionally treating a variety of health care professionals for chemical dependency, and of service on state regulatory boards and in nurses' associations. We have served on committees for impaired health care professionals. We have struggled with the language of model legislation for chemically dependent nurses, and we have helped professional associations and employers plan for the needs of chemically dependent nurses in a variety of settings. We have been consultants, expert witnesses, intervenors, monitors of abstinence, and worriers. We have lectured, testified before Congress and state legislatures, conducted research on chemical dependency in nurses, written about the issues, and planned and presented educational programs.

This issue has been a passion for us at times, as well as a source of heartbreak and exultation, of frustration, and also enormous gratification.

Through this book, we offer what we know. There is still much to learn and much to accomplish. The work is hard, challenging, misunderstood, and underfunded. We need to pool our resources and our knowledge, and to work together to overcome this dangerous and difficult problem for our colleagues, our friends, and our professions. It is our hope that this book will take us a few steps toward the solution we all seek.

Eleanor Sullivan
LeClair Bissell
Etta Williams

Acknowledgments

We wish to extend our appreciation and thanks to:

o The manuscript preparation team: Germaine Freese, research assistant; Carole Mandis, secretary; Eileen Deitcher, editorial assistant; and Sandra Sheldon, typist.

o Pharmacist Carol Bohach, who gave us valuable information on drug testing.

o The staff at Addison-Wesley Health Sciences Division, in particular, sponsoring editor Nancy Evans, production supervisor Wendy Earl, and editorial assistant Laurie Bryant.

o Our reviewers, whose constructive suggestions enhance the quality of this book: Sally Farnham, RN, MSN, California State University, Los Angeles; Patricia Green, MSW, MSN, Chair, Impaired Nurse Committee, National Nurses Society on Addictions, and member, American Nurses' Association Committee on Impaired Nursing Practice; Rick Palmisano, RN, BSN and Dawn Veatch, RN, MSN, Northwestern Memorial Hospital, Chicago; Jody Ross Yeary, PhD, MFCC, Marriage and Family Counselor, San Francisco.

And finally, we offer special thanks to the pioneers: Millicent Buxton, Rose Dilday, Barbara Ensor, Pat Green, Betty Harakal, Marty Jessup, Doris Leffler, and Nancy Miller-Cross, and to all the nurses who shared their stories with us in an attempt to "change the things we can."

CHAPTER 1

THE IMPERATIVE OF CHEMICAL DEPENDENCY MANAGEMENT FOR THE NURSING PROFESSION

INTRODUCTION: THE DEADLY DIVERSION

The use of mood-altering chemicals and the disease of chemical dependency have long been part of the human condition. Attitudes about these matters have ebbed and flowed. Today we commonly accept the notion that there are chemical solutions to most human problems. Before the advent of modern health care practices, "medicine" centered around *removing* the cause of illness; we bled and purged, cupped and leached, danced, chanted, and shook rattles to coax out the evil from the body. Now we rely on a multitude of medications we put *into* the body to restore health.

Despite our pervasive faith in drugs and medications, we also fear their potential for abuse. This fear has become particularly urgent as our society—indeed the entire world—has become increasingly interdependent. It is almost impossible to avoid responsibility for someone else's well-being; in fact, technology has made it possible for individuals to have significant impact on hundreds, thousands, even millions of others.

Drug abuse ultimately impairs a person's ability to meet personal, social, and professional responsibilities. It may be easy to ignore the addicted "street person" who seems harmless to others. However, it is less easy to feel comfortable that a nurse, a surgeon, a schoolbus driver, or an airplane pilot may be risking the lives of other people while under the influence of alcohol or another drug. Almost any addicted person has the potential to harm other people, whether by driving drunk, neglecting his/her children, or incompetently practicing a caretaking profession. Indeed, almost any job performed in an impaired condition constitutes some risk or loss to our society. Nurses working while dulled by mood-altering chemicals cannot be fully responsive to changing patient conditions, nor can they monitor patient responses to medications and treatments as skillfully.

The Throwaway Nurse Syndrome

For generations, health care employers have fired nurses whom they suspected of addiction, most often, ostensibly, for poor performance or attendance. This "throwaway nurse syndrome" did little to alleviate the true consequences of this disease. Most directly, the hospital incurs a significant financial and human cost to replace fired personnel. A study of nurses recovering from chemical dependency (Bissell & Jones, 1981) revealed that the nurses had held responsible and advanced positions; replacing such experienced nurses would be expensive. Even before the mounting shortage of nurses, estimates of the cost to replace a single registered nurse range from $1,500 (Hoffman, 1985) to $3,300 (Collins, 1984) depending on the nurse's level of education, experience, and position. Replacement costs include expenses related to advertising, recruitment, personnel fees and salaries, interviewing, selection, orientation and training, as well as overtime costs incurred during the training of the replacement nurse.

The Hidden Costs of Chemical Dependency

Long before the more obvious performance problems appear, a chemically dependent nurse may already have contributed to many "hidden" costs such as increased use of health insurance benefits, lowered productivity, increased absenteeism and tardiness, poor patient relations, poor supervisory decisions, reduced staff morale, and increased mistakes and accidents (some of which may jeopardize patient safety and lead to litigation or a damaged reputation for the institution *and* the nurse). The summary firing of one chemically dependent nurse may well inhibit an employer's ability to identify others on staff who may have drug problems, for when colleagues see this harsh response, they may be reluctant to report friends' suspected drug abuse problems. Those concerned that they may be developing a dependency problem will be even more reluctant to face the issue and are likely to invest more effort in avoiding detection if they know that being discovered means being fired and disgraced.

This does not suggest that firing is never warranted. With a clearer understanding of the nature of the disease and better knowledge of alternate approaches to interrupting its progress, most affected nurses can be helped to overcome their problems and return to work. A humane system of intervention and treatment can redeem the future for the chemically dependent nurse while significantly reducing cost and risk for health care employers. Indeed, each employee whose life is improved represents a human savings that multiplies through the years of sustained recovery (Collins, 1984). To achieve such an outcome, we must first understand the nature of the disease of chemical dependency and dispel a legacy of misinformation and myth.

UNDERSTANDING THE DISEASE

Defining Chemical Dependency

The chemical dependency field is plagued by inconsistent usage and poorly defined terms. Authors rarely describe exactly what they mean. A reviewer of the literature is easily lost in terms such as *use, abuse, misuse, dependency, addiction, polydrug, dual impairment,* and so on. Some writers apply the perjorative "abuse" to any use of a prescription drug that exceeds a physician's order. By this definition, acceptance of a single tranquilizer from a friend constitutes abuse.

The seriousness of this concept becomes clear when one reads about "drug abuse" in high school. Since the adolescents involved are underage, all drinking becomes "misuse," any episode of drunkenness equated with "abuse," and experimentation with amphetamines, marijuana, or cocaine may be reported as if the young experimenter and the serious addict were the same. A large number of minors may be harmfully involved with drugs in high school and grade school, but not all minors are dependent on drugs.

The authors prefer to avoid the term *substance abuse* because of its judgmental overtones and because it has been used in the past to refer to drugs other than alcohol, especially by those who have regarded addiction not as a primary illness but as a symptom of an external or internal emotional stressor.[1]

We use the term "chemical dependency" and sometimes the word *addiction* to refer to both physical and emotional dependency. There need not be a major physical withdrawal state when a drug is discontinued and tolerance need not be demonstrated. Adoption of that framework would identify every person having several drinks on a single evening as an addict, since one can demonstrate a mild though measurable rebound excitation after the sedation effect of alcohol is gone. Cocaine users become more sensitive with prolonged use due to a phenomenon known as "kindling," which may leave them more seizure prone than the naive user.

James Orford, a psychologist lecturing at the Maudsly Hospital in London, has said that we should measure the strength of an addiction not by whether or not a person becomes physically ill when a drug is withdrawn but, rather, by what that person will forfeit to avoid giving up the use of that drug. When cocaine, alcohol, or narcotics come before the welfare of a beloved family member, a valued career, one's life savings, one's health, even the ability to avoid jail, that is addiction.

The key to understanding addiction may be the realization that the addiction has little bearing on the legal status of a particular drug, although social and financial problems are more complex with illicit drugs.

---

[1]Some people believe "substance abuse" echoes "the mental health model" as opposed to "the Minnesota model." The latter uses the term *chemical dependency* to include all the mood-changing drugs of addiction. The Minnesota model regards dependency as the primary problem (to be addressed before other diagnosis and treatment planning occur), adopts total abstinence as the treatment goal, relies on education and redefinition of terms as part of the recovery process, and is strongly supportive of the use of mutual help groups like Alcoholics Anonymous (AA), Narcotics Anonymous (NA), and Al-Anon as supplements to treatment.

Loss of Judgment and Control

Chemical dependency involves drinking or using other drugs against what is clearly one's own best interests, at least to non-moralistic, objective outsiders. If, after drinking, judgment is so clouded that repeated arrests for driving under the influence are ruining reputation, risking lives, and incurring huge attorney's fees, it makes little difference that the drinking happens only on weekends. To continue drinking in this way reflects a loss of choice or reveals a priority system in which an abnormally high value is placed on alcohol.

Chemical dependency involves loss of control, loss of the ability to predict reliably how much one is going to drink or use on a given occasion or, if one is abstinent, when one will start again. Remember that most alcoholics are in control of most of their drinking most of the time. If every drinking or drug episode led to disaster, the consequences would be almost impossible to ignore. The truth is more complex, and the erratic nature of the results of drinking and using augment denial and rationalization. When a cocaine user has to ingest every grain before stopping a run or when an alcoholic has repeatedly vowed to stop after two or three drinks and several times is unable to do so, that is loss of control.

Compulsion to Use

Chemical dependency reflects a belief that the answer to human problems lies in finding the right medicines; that life cannot be satisfactory without the abused drugs, even though it may be rationalized that their use is only temporary. One feels *compelled* to use. The words "want" and "need" are not used interchangeably by the chemically dependent nurse. A drink or drug is *needed*, not just wanted. The nurse may describe self-loathing and distaste for her situation while simultaneously filling the glass or the syringe.

Chemical dependency rarely involves the use of only one drug. Minor tranquilizers are used to manage the insomnia and nervousness that are part of alcohol withdrawal. Amphetamines relieve depression when cocaine is unavailable. Narcotics and alcohol soften the nervous, "wired up" dysphoria some cocaine users experience. It is very easy to use a whole cafeteria of drugs, together or sequentially, and not uncommon for a nurse to acknowledge a problem with one drug, swear off it, and switch to another. There are jokes about patients who think that "alcoholism is a disease characterized by a chronic underlying Valium deficiency." The most important principle is that once chemically dependent, the nurse will not be able to use other addictive drugs safely and that this limitation is a permanent one. There are a handful of addicts who have been able to continue minimal social drinking or take an occasional tranquilizer, but the vast majority have to give up *all* of the potentially addictive drugs.

X Chemical dependency involves loss of control, compulsion to use, continued use against one's own best interests, and in spite of risk and adverse consequences, a belief in the efficacy of drugs, denial of a problem, and the need to abstain from all mood-changing, addicting drugs for permanent recovery. Physical dependency may not be a factor. Addiction should not be defined in terms of the legal status of the drugs involved. The number of nurse-users varies according to availability of the drug of choice, the law, and social trends. Alcohol is and probably will remain the most significant problem since it is inexpensive, widely available, legal and familiar, generates little upset or excitement, and is easier to ignore than diversion of other drugs.

DUAL IMPAIRMENT—PSYCHOPATHOLOGY AND ADDICTION

Chemical dependency is a primary illness; however, chemically dependent people often appear to have other psychological problems. It is frequently difficult to sort out cause and effect. For instance, alcohol is a depressant drug and anyone drinking it in large quantities and at frequent intervals is very likely to suffer from its depressive effects.

Psychiatric and Social Problems

Research (Kline & Snyder, 1985) suggests that psychopathology and alcoholism are associated and may, in some cases, presage potential chemical dependency problems. Anxiety and depression are significantly associated with alcoholism in many studies (Hasin, Endicott, & Lewis, 1985; Hesselbrock, Meyer, & Keener, 1985; Nichols, 1985; Thyer, 1986). Other emotional, family, and social problems may develop as an addiction progresses, thus clouding recognition of its primary role in their causation. Although emotional problems may affect the progression of the disease, it is essential to diagnose and treat chemical dependency *before* other psychological problems are investigated. Most problems disappear when drinking/drug taking ceases. In one study of severely depressed alcoholics (Dackis, Gold, Pottash, & Sweeney, 1986), 80% were no longer clinically depressed after two weeks of sobriety. In any case, no effective treatment is likely to occur for any other disorder while the person is actively using drugs, and even diagnosis will be extremely difficult.

Beckman (1975, 1978) reports that female alcoholics receive a psychiatric diagnosis more often than males. Since women's drinking or drug taking is more stigmatized, women may be more likely to plead psychological distress than to reveal the extent of their drug use. Thus, they are more apt to be diagnosed and treated for psychiatric disorders. Since most nurses are female, they may receive the psychiatric diagnoses commonly given to other female alcoholics. In a study of 139 chemically dependent nurses (Sullivan, 1987a), 89 subjects (64%) reported they also suffered from depression.

Psychiatric or psychological symptoms may, however, obscure recognition of the addiction problem and vice versa. Nurses whose drug use yields symptoms of anxiety or depression may be treated for those symptoms with medications that cause dependency, thus increasing drug use. Determining the nurse's correct diagnosis (or diagnoses) is the task of those expert in chemical dependency *and* in psychiatry or psychology. Timing is important, since it is virtually impossible to diagnose (or treat) psychiatric problems until drugs are removed from the equation. It is important that *both* problems be diagnosed and treated. Probably 5–10% of addicted nurses will have significant emotional problems, distinct from their chemical dependency, that will require evaluation and attention early in treatment. Chemically dependent people may also experience physical, psychological, and social problems. Heavy long-term alcohol and other drug use damages brain and body tissue and impairs their functioning. Difficulties with recent memory and new learning are very common. Ability to concentrate and to abstract are diminished.

This syndrome was apparent during a recent attempt by a major union to put recently discharged alcoholic members into a classroom situation. Fresh from treatment, the union members needed extra time before returning to the work setting with its stresses and temptations. Class placement was based on tests of previous knowledge. The students were motivated and remained sober, but they did not do well academically. Except when carefully tested for organicity, they appeared entirely normal but they were not able to learn new material. Most could, however, master new learning a few weeks or months later.

Physical Problems

Gastric and hepatic disorders, cardiovascular impairment, and neurological damage may also occur. Most of these physical problems are reversible in time. Emotionally, the addict is unable to handle the normal daily stress of marital and family relationships, which become strained and often dysfunctional. For some addicts, an active social life may center around drinking or other drug use; for others, chemical dependency leaves them increasingly isolated. Either way, social life, as well as occupational functioning, is affected. Daily activities such as parenting, PTA, or dinner with friends must be considered in the context of the need for the next drink, the next pill, the next shot, or the need to hide the truth. The physical, psychological, and social problems that develop must be addressed in treating the dependent nurse (DeSoto, O'Donnell, Alfred, & Lopes, 1985).

CHEMICAL DEPENDENCY IN NURSES

Is Nursing Different?

Chemical dependency occurs in almost every population group. We have discussed the special costs and risks that are involved when chemical dependency affects nursing practice. Are there aspects of the nursing profession that make chemical dependency a particular risk for nurses?

Stress is a natural area of inquiry. Although there is little evidence that stress itself leads to drinking and other drug use, it is still popular to examine stress-provoking professional situations. However, if stress were a reliable predictor of chemical dependency, many adults — nurses, physicians, police, air traffic controllers, single parents, movie stars, legislators, and others—would be likely candidates for chemical dependency. Stress is not a unique feature of nursing, nor of chemically dependent nurses.

The emphasis placed on drugs as valuable, useful tools of the trade is unique to nursing, pharmacy, dentistry, and medicine. Nurses, pharmacists, physicians, and dentists are taught to understand and appreciate drugs. We know how to recognize the physical signs of addiction. As professionals, we are so well informed that we sometimes begin to believe ourselves immune from the dangers of addiction. We prescribe for ourselves and for each other, and we assume we can recognize any signs of trouble. Self-medication is commonplace, and the isolated event may turn into more regular use, then compulsive use, and finally full addiction, without the user's recognition. Health care professionals have more access to dangerous narcotics—drugs more potent and lethal than are easily available to most people. And because a nurse's work involves the care and safety of vulnerable people, a professional future is at stake if a nurse becomes chemically dependent. Few other addicted professionals in our society stand to lose not only their present job, but their license to practice their profession anywhere.

No less burdensome is the emotional jeopardy that chemically dependent nurses face. Many nurses violate their own ethical principles by stealing drugs from hospital supplies or even from their patients, or they risk their patients' welfare by practicing while impaired. A nurse may be nearly overwhelmed with shame and guilt over past acts of omission or commission.

How does it happen? A nurse in California, working at a large medical center for 12 years, had risen to a position of extensive responsibility, including supervision of five intensive care units. He was liked and respected equally by those he supervised and those who supervised him. One day, after helping with an emergency in one of the units, he discovered a syringe containing a narcotic in his pocket. He was confused until he remembered that one of the other nurses had asked him to waste it. (The patient had needed only part of the dose.) He placed the syringe on his desk, intending to return it to the unit. His memory of what happened next is quite clear. He picked it up, used his stethoscope as a tourniquet, and injected the narcotic into a vein. He says it was like watching someone else, and he has no idea why he did it; curiosity is his best explanation.

His illness progressed very rapidly thereafter; he routinely stole drugs from all the units on a daily basis. Six months later the security guards, accompanied by the sheriff's department, burst into his office, arrested him, handcuffed him, and took him to jail. He heard absolutely nothing from any of the nurses with whom he had worked for 12 years.

This man has been sober for five years, but he is not working in nursing and says he is not interested in ever returning, so bitter is the memory of the arrest and the lack of caring and support demonstrated by his co-workers.

Special Populations Within the Nursing Profession

There are common denominators in the special dangers leading to chemical dependency in nurses; however, it must also be stressed that nurses are individuals. Each has a unique set of personal, family, health, and sociocultural characteristics that play important roles in their respective attitudes toward the use of alcohol and other drugs.

It has been suggested (Haack & Harford, 1984; Perrin, 1983) that nurses and social workers are more likely than other professionals to be children of alcoholics. As children, these caretakers may have accepted the role of "family heroine," assuming responsibility for a parent who could not adequately meet family obligations. This child cared for the younger children and nursed the family through hangovers and other illnesses. Children accepting this role also tend to get good grades and to please adults. They use their success to show that the family is really all right. Children of alcoholics often marry alcoholics. Further, children of alcoholics are at greater risk of becoming chemically dependent themselves (Goodwin, 1981). This profile may not apply to nurses in general; however, it *has* been documented that there is a greater incidence of alcoholism in the nuclear families of chemically dependent nurses (Bissell & Haberman, 1984). "Co-dependency" (the set of maladaptive and/or immature responses, behaviors, and feelings experienced by someone living with an actively chemically dependent person) is a problem for many nurses with chemically dependent spouses.

Bissell and Haberman's 1984 report on 407 recovered alcoholics, 73% of whom worked in health care, revealed that 36% had at least one alcoholic parent. A further breakdown of this statistic showed that 41% of the women and 29% of the men reported an alcoholic parent. A group of physicians, attorneys, and dentists (all but five were men) was similar, with 29%, 27%, and 24% respectively. More nurses than college women and social workers reported alcoholic parents, 46%,

39%, and 38% respectively. Within this group, 100 nurses, 56 college women (not in health care), and 60% of the social workers were female. A recent report by Bissell and Skorina (1987) on 100 alcoholic female physicians and medical students revealed that 56% of them had an alcoholic parent. The same patterns are emerging from Bissell and Skorina's studies of alcoholic nuns and psychologists.

If we can document the caretaking function of "family heroine," what of the good grades, the high achievement? When Bissell and Haberman (1984) examined class standing at professional school graduation, all the professional groups they interviewed showed a marked tendency to graduate in the upper or middle third of their classes. This information was not as definitive for nurses as for the other groups, since many of the nurses—particularly diploma school graduates— were not given their class rank. Furthermore, some graduating classes were too small for the relevant comparison. The pattern appears the same, however. Brennan (1983) interviewed 50 abstinent alcoholic nurses in New Jersey (49 white, 1 black; 47 women, 3 men). Twenty-eight (56%) had at least one alcoholic parent; 39 (86%) had ranked in the top third of their nursing class. Reed (1986) reports on 26 subjects, 5 of them male and 12 with addiction to drugs other than alcohol. Nine (35%) had a chemically dependent parent and 69% were in the upper third of their classes. Of Jaffe's (1982) group of 16, 6 held master's degrees.

All of the above studies involved face-to-face interviews with nurses in one stage or another of recovery. Sullivan (1987b) studied a larger population and included a comparison group of 522 nurses who did not admit to an alcohol or drug problem. Her respondents form the largest group of chemical dependents studied thus far: 139 registered nurses, of whom 122 (87%) were women and 17 (13%) were men. In this study, both groups (who completed a direct mail questionnaire) reported success in school: 64% graduated in the upper fourth of their nursing classes. Sibling rank was also the same in both groups, with 70% being first or second born. Differences were evident, however, in family background. In the chemically dependent nurse sample, 48% indicated that family circumstances forced them to assume parental roles during childhood compared to only 22% of the control group. Heavy drinking in the parental home was reported by 32% of the chemically dependent nurses and only 10% of the comparison group. An alcoholic family member was identified by 62% of the dependent sample, but by only 28% of the comparison group.

Gender Differences

Since nursing is largely a woman's profession, the chemically dependent nurse is more likely to be female than male. There is, however, some indication that male nurses are more likely to be chemically dependent. The percentage of men in nursing who are brought to the attention of disciplinary bodies for addiction problems is higher than for women (Sullivan, 1987a). (It must be stressed again, however, that the overall percentage of addiction problems reaching a disciplinary body is quite small.) In the general public, there are more alcoholic men than alcoholic women. There are also more men known to be addicted to cocaine, marijuana, and parenteral narcotics. Data suggest that women may outnumber men in tranquilizer, sedative, and diet pill dependency. However, since ready access to a more sophisticated spectrum of drugs is increased in the health care field, it is unclear whether gender differences in drug use patterns would apply to nurses.

Since only 3% of nurses are male, we would expect 6% of those disciplined for alcoholism problems to be men, which would reflect the accepted finding that men in any profession are twice as likely to be alcoholic as women. Nurse support groups frequently comment, however, that more than 15% of their members are men. Formal data are not currently available, but informal reports are common and it is our impression that men are indeed overrepresented. We learned recently that more men than women were being monitored after treatment in one midwestern state.

There may be, in general, a greater readiness to identify men as alcoholic. Or perhaps men in nursing are still rare and are thus highly visible. Colleagues tend to be aware of them and interested in them, so perhaps problems are more quickly noticed and reported. Men in nursing, like women in medicine, have formed a small minority within their chosen profession. They have not been fully included in the "old girl" network. They have been somewhat isolated from peers and have had to face questions about sexual orientation and motives for choosing a career long perceived as exclusively for women.

The experience of employee assistance programs in non–health care fields has demonstrated that even when adjusted for age, total workforce numbers, and the varying expected rates of alcoholism in each gender group, women remain much less likely than men to be referred by others for drinking or other drug problems. They are, however, more likely to seek help for themselves. Perhaps the same phenomenon exists among nurses as well. Perhaps if nurses had a safe place to go for help they would seek it on their own, rather than fear censure.

Choice of Drugs

While the choice of addictive drugs depends greatly on individual circumstances, there are some patterns of drug use that reflect drug availability at specific hospital job assignments. Nurse anesthetists, along with anesthesiologists, are said to be at particularly high risk, although no convincing data exist to support this assumption. Narcotics such as Demerol®(meperidine) are widely available in hospital units, whereas narcotics like fentanyl are more likely to be used in and around the operating or delivery room. Not surprisingly, anesthesiologists and nurse anesthetists are most likely to be addicted to fentanyl.[2] Demerol use has been linked to those working in areas in which it is rather easily available: surgery, anesthesia, emergency, and intensive care units.

A more uncommon problem, the abuse of volatile gases is linked with dentists' offices or operating rooms. An anesthesiologist describes bending over his patient, cautiously lifting the mask while pretending to adjust it, and inhaling deeply. He did this repeatedly until he lost consciousness in the operating room while sharing penthrane with a patient. "The patient was waking up and I was out cold," he reported.

It is clear that diversion of hospital drugs is linked to their availability, but cause and effect are not always obvious. Did the narcotics use begin when the nurse found them accessible, or did the already chemically dependent nurse manipulate the job assignments to obtain drugs more easily? Was the drug use provoked by the "high stress" levels characteristic of acute care nursing? (And is the stress in acute care really more intense than, for instance, in oncology or on AIDS units?)

Changes in work site appear to reflect the progression of the illness. Chemically dependent nurses often move gradually from positions of

---

[2]Fentanyl is more rapidly metabolized than Demerol and most other powerful opiates, hence it vanishes from the urine more rapidly and is harder to detect in drug screens.

great responsibility to a phase called "job shrinkage." In this phase duties are performed quite adequately, but the "extras" slowly diminish. The nurse participates in fewer committees, decreases attendance at professional and semi-social events, and does not attend workshops or give presentations as often. Plausible explanations, such as family obligations or health problems, are given. The nurse becomes less available. Then a new pattern is established. The nurse does only what is required, and when work performance begins to suffer, commonly the nurse will resign or seek reassignment "before the ax falls." The new position may be a conscious move to a position of less pressure, less responsibility, less visibility, or less supervision.

Since so many nurses (97%) are women, it has been relatively easy for those with chemical dependency problems to explain gradual job changes in terms of obligations to husband and children. The nurse can move downward, one step at a time, from charge nurse to staff nurse to night nurse to temporary services. Each change in itself is not very dramatic.

Choice of drugs is not a simple matter of job assignment and access to narcotics. Many chemically dependent nurses are addicted to alcohol, prescription drugs, or "street drugs." Many never try narcotics or cocaine; some experiment once or twice. Many have multiple addictions. Bissell and Jones's 1981 study of 100 alcoholic women nurses reported that 14 were also addicted to narcotics and an additional 21 were addicted to other mood-altering drugs. Many more reported use of other drugs but without addiction. In Sullivan's 1987 study of 139 chemically dependent nurses (including 17 men) only 43% reported alcohol addiction alone; 55% reported addiction to narcotics; 37% reported use of "street drugs." Other studies (Kelley, 1985; Levine, Preston, & Lipscomb, 1974; Poplar, 1969; Reed, 1986) confirm nurses' addiction to multiple drugs.

Nurses are individuals outside their jobs, and their choice of drugs and patterns of use also reflect age and American social trends. Recent papers on drug use by pharmacists, physicians, pharmacy students, and medical students (McAuliffe, Rohman, Santangelo, Feldman, Magnuson, Sobol, & Weissman, 1986; McAuliffe, Santangelo, Gingras, Rohman, Sobol, & Magnuson, 1987) clearly reflect this. It is believed that the children of the sixties use marijuana and psychedelics more than their parents. Today, widespread social use of cocaine is reported in all the newspapers. Younger nurses are more likely to smoke marijuana and snort cocaine than older ones. Older nurses are more likely to use alcohol, amphetamines, soporifics, and tranquilizers. Nurses are nurses, but they also belong to their own generation, with its fads, its taste in music, its style of dancing, and, in many cases, its choice of drugs.

THE PREVALENCE OF CHEMICAL DEPENDENCY IN THE NURSING PROFESSION

Despite the special characteristics of the nursing profession, there is no evidence that a nursing education guarantees special protection against alcoholism, nor does it put one at special risk. There is no reliable estimate of the actual numbers of nurses who suffer from chemical dependency, although the existing approaches to determine prevalence do suggest certain patterns. The following approaches have been used to determine prevalence.

Surveys

Because alcoholism and other addictions still carry a stigma, particularly for women, a survey on alcohol or drug use may not yield a representative sample or truthful response. Denial—not just to others but to oneself—is a hallmark of chemical dependency. Often the alcoholic is the last to know that a problem exists, and what cannot be acknowledged to oneself is impossible to share with others. Chemical dependency cannot be mentioned, and questions about it must therefore be indirect.

When professional colleagues are surveyed about their awareness of others with alcohol or drug problems, it becomes apparent that most recognized cases are identified by a relatively small number of people. Those who have recovered from alcoholism or have worked in the chemical dependency area can usually identify alcoholic colleagues easily. Others who work in the same hospitals and are in contact with the same individuals commonly remain unaware of such problems. The result is that the estimated numbers of chemically dependent nurses are a reflection of the skills of the observer rather than of the external reality.

Licensure Sanctions

A less subjective approach to determining prevalence in the profession involves examination of the activities of regulatory agencies and disciplinary groups. Every state has a licensing board for the nursing profession and the chemical dependency cases handled by such boards can be tallied. This information will become more useful as record-keeping uniformity increases and case findings are organized. At present, however, there is tremendous variation among different states, with some boards energetically seeking out professionals in trouble and others ignoring all but the most spectacular cases.

Further, we do not know what percentage of chemically dependent nurses come to the attention of a regulatory board. A report from the National Council of State Boards of Nursing (1980–1981) indicates that two-thirds of disciplinary actions against nurses' licenses are related to the "use, abuse or misuse" of alcohol or controlled substances. A more recent survey of 44 state boards of nursing revealed that 67% of cases handled by the boards were related to substance abuse (see Appendix H). However, many recovering nurses report that, although they drank alcohol or used drugs on the job, they were not reported to the state board and that their nursing licenses were never in jeopardy. We must assume, then, that most chemically dependent nurses will *not* have a formal record of chemical dependency. The mechanisms of disciplinary actions of state boards are discussed further in Chapter 8.

A study of alcoholic male physicians and female nurses in the 1970s (Bissell & Haberman, 1984) revealed that only 7% of 97 male physicians and 3% of 100 female registered nurses actually lost licenses. Of 49 dentists, 50 social workers, and 55 attorneys, none lost licenses or were disbarred. A more recent study of 100 alcoholic female physicians and medical students (Bissell & Skorina, 1987) revealed that, despite the recent rapid growth of awareness of physicians' impairment from alcohol and/or drugs, only 5% of these women lost licenses. Of the male physicians studied in the 1970s, 34% never received sanctions for their drinking or drug abuse. It is significant that as many as 58% of the women studied years later escaped sanctions. The sanctions in these studies included even an informal admonition by a colleague. Over 75% of the alcoholic physicians and nurses studied in the 1970s reported that they had escaped formal sanctions, even though 12% of the nurses, 14% of the male physicians, and 17% of the female physicians were addicted to narcotics as well. Most of the physicians also reported use of alcohol during working hours.

It is clear from these studies that some problems are more likely than others to be reported to various professional regulatory boards. Regulatory boards for psychologists and social workers, for instance, are inclined to ignore addictions altogether and are more likely to review or revoke licenses if patients are being sexually exploited by a therapist, particularly if the therapist is male. Nurses, pharmacists, and physicians are more likely to be reported for diverting (stealing) drugs from work, particularly cocaine or narcotics. They are unlikely to be disciplined for drinking or using marijuana or other street drugs or for using non-narcotic prescription tranquilizers, soporifics, or stimulants. Apparently the legality of the drug of choice, its classification as a controlled substance, and its source are aspects more likely to provoke disciplinary action than impairment of job performance.

Population in Treatment

The prevalence of chemical dependency in nurses is also evidenced by the numbers who receive treatment. According to astute and credible observers, both nurses and physicians are overrepresented in treatment populations. In 1968, Glatt wrote that the number of physicians and nurses admitted for alcoholism at his facility near London far exceeded their proportional representation in the total population. Murray (1976) also found a disproportionate number of physicians admitted for cirrhosis to a hospital in Scotland, compared with a comparable group of equally affluent and educated white male attorneys.

Other researchers have noted the disproportionate numbers of doctors and nurses in treatment and concluded that they may be at unusually high risk. These observations about treatment populations may tell only part of the story however. When alcoholics in recovery in other occupational groups were asked about their hospital admission experience during the drinking years, it became apparent that health care professionals were indeed more likely to enter residential treatment (Bissell & Haberman, 1984). The number of reported admissions for inpatient chemical dependency treatment included an average of 6.3 admissions each for male physicians, 4.1 admissions for nurses, and 3.2 admissions for dentists. Attorneys were admitted an average of 1.9

times, social workers 2.4 times, and college women 2.6 times. Assuming that alcoholism in a nurse or physician is no more serious physically than for those in other professions, it is likely that the difference in treatment populations reflects the subjects' attitudes about seeking treatment rather than the prevalence of disease itself. Thus, health care professionals may be more likely to seek or accept hospital care than others.

Correlations with Other Illnesses

When another illness accompanies chemical dependency, we can use its prevalence to estimate the prevalence of chemical dependency. For instance, pancreatitis or cirrhosis commonly accompanies alcoholism. The best known formula for such a correlation, the Jellinek Formula, examines the amount of cirrhosis in a population, assumes that a known proportion of cirrhotics are alcoholic, then extrapolates the number of alcoholics in that population. This formula assumes that the cirrhosis numbers are accurate, that the considered population is not at unusual risk for liver disease, and that the proportion of alcoholic cirrhotics is accurately known. The use of this formula may indeed yield useful information even though Jellinek's work has been strongly challenged. Unfortunately, however, even if we accept Jellinek's approach, we lack the necessary data for nurses. Statistics on deaths from cirrhosis in nurses do exist but are disputed. Most data on alcoholism and cirrhosis in the general population have been collected for men rather than women, a recurrent problem in research on addictive illness. In addition, a liver that has been damaged by hepatitis is more prone to cirrhosis, and health care workers are known to be at increased risk for hepatitis.

Educated Guesses

Despite the lack of nurse-specific data, we can make educated guesses based on our general knowledge of chemical dependency. About 10% of American adult males and 5% of women are or will become alcoholic. Since nursing remains predominantly a woman's profession, we can infer that between 5–6% of nurses are or will be alcoholic (if the profession itself does not increase or decrease the risk). Estimates of nurses affected by addiction to prescription drugs and/or narcotics are even less reliable. The National Institute on Drug Abuse estimates that 1–2% of Americans are drug dependent, and that roughly 500,000 are addicted to narcotics. Exact numbers are lacking; however, it appears that health care professionals are more likely to use narcotics than lay people because of their easy access. Many researchers suspect there may also be a greater risk in the health care professions of prescription drug addiction or involvement with cocaine.

In considering the various approaches to determining prevalence of chemical dependency in nurses, there is evidence of certain patterns. Although the data are not conclusive, an awareness of the factors that may play an important role in a nurse's potential risk of chemical dependency is important.

WHY IS THE PROBLEM OBSCURED?

The Conspiracy of Silence

While our ignorance about the prevalence of chemical dependency in nurses is, in part, due to lack of sufficient data, much has also been written about the so-called conspiracy of silence: Professionals appear deliberately to cover up for their peers. It has even been suggested that this reluctance to expose the problem within a profession is rooted in an individual's own chemical dependency problem. These personal fears for self and colleagues do play a role in covering up chemical dependency in the health care professions, but the greatest problem may be sheer ignorance about the disease.

Despite their professional training, many health care professionals feel poorly equipped to address chemical dependency problems—either in themselves or others. We recently conducted an unpublished survey of approximately 300 health care professionals, including 100 nurses, some of whom have been chemically dependent and some of whom have been closely involved with other chemically dependent people. Respondents were asked if they felt their education had prepared them to recognize and deal with addiction. The response was an almost unanimous "no." And many respondents felt compelled to add exclamation marks and unsolicited comments.

Educational Factors

Nursing education must cover a great deal of content and comprehensive skill development in a relatively short time—as little as two years in an associate degree program. A graduate must pass a rigorous two-day licensure examination, which currently includes few questions on chemical dependency. Most nursing schools are hard-pressed to cover the content that they know *will* be covered on the licensure examination. Education related to chemical dependency generally includes detoxification techniques and the toxic effects of excessive use of drugs. Few schools present information on alcoholism and other addictions as primary diseases. At the master's level, study focuses on a specialty role in a clinical area, in management, or in education. Doctoral study concentrates on research, theory development, and nursing education.

Since so little is taught about addiction, nurses often are not aware that there *is* a pertinent body of knowledge about addictive diseases. Hence they (and other health care professionals) either believe they *do* know everything there is to know about the disease, or they believe that such knowledge is not relevant to their practice.

Once licensed, a nurse is expected to keep abreast of the latest information and to keep clinical skills up to date. When selecting continuing education programs, unless the content is clearly relevant to their work or their lives, they are likely to neglect addiction education. Other topics may seem more important in their daily work than chemical dependency.

Even medical schools commonly neglect the study of chemical dependency (Pokorney & Solomon, 1983) and may settle for vague warnings about prescribing drugs for oneself and one's family or friends. Health care employers likewise seldom include the disease process, signs, and symptoms in their orientation or inservice training for nurses, although they are likely to mention institutional policies on theft of hospital property (including drugs).

Despite the constraints on content about chemical dependency in nursing education, it is imperative that curricula be improved. A model curriculum for nursing education is offered in Appendix A. Chapter 11 contains specific recommendations for improving nursing education in chemical dependency. Nurses must be able to recognize chemical dependency as a factor in their patients' illnesses and to understand the personal risks associated with this devastating disease.

ORGANIZED NURSING RESPONSES

The Roman Catholic Church long ago took action to identify and assist its alcoholic priests, but the legal and health care professions lagged far behind. Disciplines which were composed largely of women reacted more slowly than male-dominated professions, and even the latter were slow to identify and refer female colleagues. Sometimes women were excluded altogether. In many cases, attention was focused on prolonged residential treatment for individuals who were an embarrassment to their peers. In some cases, the emphasis appears to have been more on hiding the problem than on rehabilitation. In 1975 the American Medical Association (AMA) sponsored its first national conference on the "Disabled Doctor." Initially worried about public response to any admission of physician addiction, the Association was much encouraged by the understanding and positive reception of the press. Evidently it was clear that continued cover-up would be perceived as less laudable than forthright attempts to resolve a problem.

Since its 1975 meeting, the AMA has held similar conferences every two years, the most recent of which included a full spectrum of health care disciplines. The AMA also publishes the *Impaired Physician* newsletter and provides back-up services for state committees. Today almost every state medical association has an assistance program for chemically dependent physicians.

Organized nursing trailed the AMA by a decade in holding its first national conference on the impaired nurse in Kansas City in 1985 (American Nurses' Association, 1985).[3] In 1980 the Ohio State Nurses Association brought the question of addicted nurses before the American Nurses' Association (ANA) House of Delegates. At the biennial meeting of the organization later that year in Houston, a resolution was

---

[3]Emory University held the "First National Symposium on the Impaired Nurse" in 1983 with subsequent symposiums held annually.

meeting of the organization later that year in Houston, a resolution was
introduced by the ANA Division of Psychiatric and Mental Health
Nursing Practice and the Commission on Economic and General
Welfare for an Assistance Program for Nurses Impaired by Mental
Disorders or Chemical Abuse. It was defeated. Later that year the
division appointed a nursing task force on Addictions and Psychological Dysfunctions. Surrounded by a sea of plastic buttons saying, "Help,
Don't Hide," the ANA finally adopted a policy statement that was
reintroduced in 1982 as "Resolution 5." Treatment was to be offered
prior to disciplinary action for chemical dependency or emotional illness. (See Appendix B for complete text of the resolution.)

Following the adoption of Resolution #5, the American Nurses'
Association Board of Directors appointed a task force of members from
the ANA Division of Psychiatric and Mental Health Nursing Practice,
the National Nurses Society on Addiction (NNSA), and the Drug and
Alcohol Nursing Association (DANA), to address the problem of
addiction in the profession. This task force developed a monograph
describing the problem and presenting information to assist state
nurses' associations in setting up assistance programs for chemically
dependent nurses (American Nurses' Association, 1984). The task
force continues to collect data and reports annually on the status of
such programs. Recently, the ANA Board of Directors appointed a permanent committee to continue data collection and to make recommendations for further action, although as we go to press the
funding for this committee is in doubt.

Specialty organizations for addiction in nursing now exist. In addition to addressing the professional concerns of nurses practicing in
the area of chemical dependency, they also assist with nurses' chemical
dependency problems. In addition, several position papers on chemical
dependency in nursing have been published (see Appendix D).

Regardless of our present inability to assess the number of nurses
lost to alcoholism and other drug dependency, we know it is significant.
We also know that more can be done to improve the situation and that
efforts to do so are already underway on many different levels of various
disciplines. A closer look at some of these actions as well as the special
challenges to nursing may help us design responses that meet the needs
of the profession more completely.

CHAPTER 2

IDENTIFYING THE CHEMICALLY DEPENDENT NURSE

SEEING IS NOT BELIEVING: DENIAL OF THE PROBLEM

Identification of a chemically dependent nurse may be difficult. The primary symptom of addictive illness is denial, a denial so profound that the addicted person truly does not see and believe what may be obvious to others. In fact, many addicts are not convinced of their chemical dependency, despite overwhelming evidence. They may acknowledge their impaired behavior, and even their use of alcohol or other drugs, while denying their drug dependency.

Common Denial Mechanisms

When discovered using alcohol and other drugs, the nurse may offer elaborate excuses. Common explanations include fatigue, use of cough syrup or antihistamines (explaining the odor of alcohol or appearance of drunkenness), or emotional stress (death in the family, marital troubles, ill child). A nurse may proclaim, "I've never done this before," and describe the situation as an isolated incident.

The problem may also be denied by colleagues, friends, and family, who find it difficult to accept that someone they know could be alcoholic or addicted to other drugs. Observers may notice sporadic heavy drinking or drug experimentation. Perhaps a temporary stress is thought to be the cause of the "incident." Everyone, including the addict, believes that time, patience, and understanding will resolve the problem.

Even when the problem can no longer be dismissed as temporary, denial by friends and associates may continue. To relieve their own sense of responsibility for delaying intervention, they seek "explanations" for the drug use, like back pain, headaches, or depression.

Denial and Job Termination

If deteriorating job performance leads to dismissal, employers often attribute the termination to other causes rather than confront the real issue. Obvious though it may be, alcohol or other drug use may never be mentioned . One nurse reports that she was found unconscious on the restroom floor with a needle in her thigh and she was fired for "being regularly late returning from lunch."

Even the regulatory system inadvertently encourages deception. In some states, if an employer fires a nurse for chemical dependency, the employer is required by law to report the nurse to the board of nursing. Most other reasons for termination need not be reported. It is easy to perpetuate the deception by firing nurses for reasons other than drug use.

Denial Among Nurses

The denial syndrome is common in all addictive illness, however, there are additional factors which may strengthen denial and weaken recognition of addiction in nurses. One factor is the social stigma against female addiction that prevails in this society. In a profession dominated by women, addicted nurses often embrace this stigma. They (and their colleagues) are often reluctant to admit to dependency problems even when denial has clearly worn thin.

Women (and nurses) traditionally have been rewarded for passivity, neatness, kindness, and obedience. Heavy drinking and other drug use are perceived as aggressive, masculine behaviors particularly unacceptable to women. There is thus more pressure to conceal drug use, and less likelihood that it will be discovered by others.

Chemical dependence in nurses is also likely to be overlooked due to common misconceptions and assumptions about nurses and addictive illnesses. Despite the fact that alcoholism has been officially designated a primary disease by the AMA, health care professionals and the lay public tend to view most alcohol and drug use as a matter of personal choice, manageable by willpower. Nurses are expected to exhibit control. They are expected to stay cool through disaster, calming other staff, patients, and relatives. As long as the addicted nurse can maintain this facade, other questionable behaviors may go unnoticed. When control is strongly valued in a profession, loss of control is particularly upsetting and frightening. Chemical dependency clearly demonstrates a loss of control.

Another factor that inhibits recognition of addiction in nurses and other health care professionals is educational background and the socialization process in the workplace. Nurses and doctors are taught to perceive medication as good and desirable and to administer it accordingly. They may fail to question each other's drug use, mistakenly assuming that all health care professionals are knowledgeable about the effects and the addiction potential of alcohol and other drugs.

The knowledge and training of health care professionals may, in fact, contribute to the denial of their own disease. They are trained to recognize the physical symptoms of addiction. If physical symptoms are absent, there is a temptation to wait for evidence of physical dependency or even to deny that the drugs used are addictive. (Physical addiction is not a prominent feature of stimulant drugs like cocaine and amphetamines.) By the time physical dependency is a factor, denial strengthens as the notion of life without the drug becomes inconceivable.

How Nurses Conceal Addictions

A paradox of denial is the conscious effort the addicted person expends on concealing the use of drugs while continuing to deny addiction. The alcohol or other drug dependent will try to maintain a normal physical appearance and an acceptable work performance for as long as possible. Many nurses make an extra effort to be well groomed. Uniforms may be spotless. Despite trembling hands, nails are trimmed and clean.

Enormous effort goes into job performance, in an attempt to make up for minor lapses. In fact, recovered nurses often report significant career success during the disease progression (Bissell & Jones, 1981).

One nurse, who was completing her doctoral dissertation, had been treated over the years for a variety of physical problems (migraine, ulcers, and tendonitis). As these problems exacerbated, her physicians prescribed tranquilizers, analgesics, and narcotics. And as her pain increased, she escalated her dosages. Her physician husband wrote prescriptions for additional drugs *they* decided she needed. A respiratory arrest resulted in hospitalization, diagnosis, and treatment. Ten years later she is teaching in a large university school of nursing.

Methods of disguising drug use vary with the specific drug(s): alcohol, legally or illegally-obtained therapeutic drugs, or illegal "street" drugs.

Prescribed Drugs

Prescription of therapeutic drugs is controlled by law. Only physicians, veterinarians, and dentists are allowed to prescribe mood-altering drugs such as amphetamines, barbiturates, tranquilizers, and narcotics. Addicted nurses often visit physicians with real or fictitious medical or emotional problems and ask for medication. A nurse's understanding of symptomatology makes it relatively easy to describe fictitious symptoms and convince the physician to prescribe the desired drug. The physician may assume that the nurse is aware of the dangers of addiction and has sufficient self-control to avoid misuse. The chemically dependent nurse may visit a number of physicians to obtain multiple prescriptions for the drug of addiction. A nurse living in an urban area said she saw over 60 physicians, only two of whom refused to prescribe for her. Many nurses obtain "hallway prescriptions" from unsuspecting physician friends. Nurses working for physicians report that sometimes they were given presigned prescription blanks to fill out as they wished.

Hospital Drugs

Addicted nurses who divert hospital drugs for their own use usually employ three methods: drug substitution, false record keeping, or theft.

With drug substitution, the entire container of medication, such as a tubex of meperidine (Demerol®), may be replaced with a container of water or saline. Or the drug may be siphoned out, either partially or completely, and substituted with water or saline. Ingenious methods are used to conceal the substitution. For example, a razor may be used to cut a slit in a box of tubexes. The drug substitution takes place and an altered tubex is replaced with no obvious evidence of tampering.

Falsification of patients' or narcotics records is another method of diverting hospital drugs for personal use. The nurse may chart a full dosage that was, in fact, partially given or not given at all. Or the patient may be given a substitute drug. The nurse may sign out unused drugs, report breakage or spillage of diverted drugs, or report frequent medication errors. One nurse expressed amazement that the highly selective nature of her clumsiness was never questioned. She repeatedly reported that she spilled meperidine, while she never broke a tubex of a phenothiazine drug.

Nurses also steal narcotic and non-narcotic drugs. They may take medications that are left unattended at the patient's bedside, in intensive care units, or in surgery. Leftover doses of non-narcotic drugs are particularly accessible after patient's discharge or from stock suppliers. Nurses may take drugs in the brief moments following the drug supply accounting by changing shifts, thus causing confusion as to when the drugs were taken. They may take an entire allotment of a drug sent from the pharmacy, including the signout sheet, thus making the disappearance look like an accounting error. The nurse may take medication left in discarded tubexes. One nurse became expert at confiscating drugs from addicted patients. He volunteered to take the confiscated drugs to the hospital pharmacist for destruction, but the drugs never reached the pharmacy. In another case, a nurse anesthetist reported that he asked drug company salesmen to send samples of controlled drugs *to his home* and they did so with no questions asked!

Alcohol and "Street" Drugs

Since the purchase of alcohol is legal for adults, and the acquisition of illegal "street" drugs like cocaine or marijuana is not generally transacted at the nurse's workplace, attempts to *acquire* these drugs do not provide observable clues to an addiction problem. If the nurse uses the drug at the workplace, it is usually done in a private office or in the restroom. The drug may be concealed in personal belongings or clothing. Even if the drug is not used at the workplace, the addicted nurse must attempt to conceal its adverse effects on job performance or appropriate behavior. Arriving at work with alcohol on one's breath may be considered poor judgment, but it is generally not a crime. Most hospitals have no written policy about drinking at lunch, even when patients must be cared for in the afternoon. As long as performance remains intact, there may be no obvious direct evidence of alcohol dependency. However, there are specific signs and symptoms that become more evident as the disease progresses.

Drug Procurement for Others

A nurse who diverts drugs is not always an addict, but may be taking them to give to others. Most commonly, nurses divert drugs to a family member or friend who is in pain and whom they believe is undermedicated. This is a common symptom of "co-dependency": the destructive behavior of people closely involved with a chemical dependent.

A recent study by the Connecticut Department of Consumer Protection (DaDalt, 1986) reports a 5% increase over a ten-year period in the number of nurses diverting drugs for someone else's use. In the 18–25-year-old group of nurses, the percentages increased from 0% to 26%. It should be noted, however, that since denial is so integral to this disease, a chemically dependent nurse confronted about drug diversion is apt to attribute the diversion to someone else's needs. To assess this possibility accurately, one must be aware of the various other signs and symptoms of addiction, which are outlined later in this chapter.

The following story illustrates the phenomenon of drug diversion for others. One nurse's teenage son became addicted to drugs while living at home and attending college. He stole both money and drugs from her over a period of many months. After an angry confrontation, she agreed to continue to bring home drugs and administer them to him herself. The plan was to taper him off at home and avoid the public embarrassment of detoxification in a hospital. Three months later the "tapering off" was still in progress; in fact, the total daily use had increased. By now the nurse was too frightened to seek outside help for fear her role in the situation would be revealed. The boy was playing on her fear of what might happen to him, as well as her fear of his reprisal should she refuse him more drugs. He threatened to kill himself and

warned that he might be sent to jail for stealing money and/or drugs.
Eventually she contacted Al-Anon and ended her own and her son's
destructive behaviors.

SIGNS AND SYMPTOMS OF ADDICTION

As tolerance for a drug develops, the user may appear normal as dosages
increase. With continual use, obvious signs and symptoms may not be
evident. Lack of knowledge regarding the more subtle, early symptoms
of the disease makes timely recognition of the problem difficult.
Changes may occur over a prolonged period. Friends and colleagues
may not recognize the significance of early symptoms until after the
disease has caused serious consequences such as accidents, drunk
driving arrests, job loss, or physical illness. Gradual changes in job
performance usually occur as well. Basic job performance may not
change appreciably but, as was discussed in Chapter 1, the "extras" are
increasingly neglected. Minimum expectations are met, but the job
shrinks. The nurse may no longer be trusted by colleagues to handle
important jobs or to assume additional tasks. The former bright light
has dimmed, although it may not have flickered discernibly.
    A single sign or symptom does not necessarily indicate chemical
dependency, but there are early patterns to watch for—especially in
combination with other symptoms.

Background Indicators

Background indicators include:

o Family history of alcoholism or drug abuse

o History of frequent change of work site, in the same or other
   institutions

o Prior medical history requiring pain control

o Prior reputation as conscientious and responsible employee

Behavioral Signs

Behavioral signs include:

o Increasing isolation from colleagues, friends, and family

o Frequent complaints of marital and family problems

o Frequent reports of illness, minor accidents, and emergencies

o Complaints from others about the person's alcohol/drug use and/or poor work performance

o Evidence of blackouts

o Mood swings, irritability, depression, or suicide threats and/or attempts (which may be caused by accidental overdose)

o Strong interest in patients' pain control, the narcotics cabinet, and use of pain control medications

o Frequent trips to the bathroom or other unexplained, brief absences

o Request for night shifts

o Social avoidance of staff; eating alone; isolation

o Elaborate or inadequate excuses for tardiness or absence, including long lunch hours or use of sick leave immediately after days off

o Difficulty meeting schedules and deadlines

o Illogical or sloppy charting

Physical Symptoms

Physical symptoms include:

o Shakiness, tremors of hands

○ Slurred speech

○ Watery eyes, dilated or constricted pupils

○ Diaphoresis

○ Unsteady gait

○ Runny nose

○ Nausea, vomiting, diarrhea

○ Weight loss or gain

○ Increasing carelessness about personal appearance

Narcotics Discrepancies

Nurse managers and staff should suspect the probability of drug diversion if any of the following occur:

○ Frequently incorrect narcotics counts

○ Apparent alteration of narcotics vials

○ Increased number of patient reports of pain medication ineffectiveness

○ Discrepancy between patient reports and hospital records of pain medication (eg, patient reports he takes pain medication only during the day, records indicate nighttime administration as well)

○ Discrepancies in physician's orders, progress notes, and narcotics records

○ Large amounts of narcotics wasted

○ Numerous corrections on narcotics records

O Erratic patterns of narcotics discrepancies (these may be timed with the addicted nurse's work schedule)

O Significant variation in quantity of drugs required on a unit

When any of these patterns emerge, the possibility of drug diversion should be investigated. Any sign of drug diversion must be considered a danger signal. The observer may be inclined to dismiss initial signals, but they must not be ignored. Further investigation is in order. Can a particular nurse be connected with any of the events? Who was on duty when the narcotics counts were off? Who was working when most of the wastage occurred? Which nurse reported much of the wastage? Did anyone else actually witness the drug spillage, or was the reporting nurse's word simply accepted? One or two nurses can usually be identified as the apparent source of drug diversions. The key is to recognize the signs.

One intensive care unit nurse exchanged water-filled tubexes with morphine- or meperidine-filled tubexes kept at the patients' bedsides. As her addiction progressed she became careless. One day she made the switch in the presence of another nurse, who was so astounded at what she *thought* she saw that she took some time to realize she should contact her supervisor. Even the supervisor doubted the alleged occurrence (McCaun, 1986).

Additional Signs and Symptoms

Additional signs and symptoms specific to a nurse who may be abusing narcotic drugs include:

O Rapid mood change from irritation to depression to euphoria

O Use of long-sleeved clothing continuously, even in warm weather

O Change in work schedule

O Appearance on the unit on days off

O Request of assignment that facilitates access to drugs

o Disappearance into the restroom immediately after accessing narcotics cabinet

As outlined above, there are many early warning signs of growing
chemical dependency. Our first hurdle is attitude. We must overcome
preconceptions about nurses, about women, and about health care
professionals. We must resist the tendency to deny the evidence, to
overlook warning signals. An understanding of signs and symptoms
and alertness to their presence will help identify a chemical dependency problem early. Once the problem is recognized, intervention
must be carefully planned. Intervention strategies are discussed in the
following chapter.

CHAPTER 3

INTERVENTION

REMOVING THE WEB OF DENIAL

When colleagues, family, or friends realize that a nurse indeed has a chemical dependency problem, the nurse usually will persist in denying the situation. A variety of serious problems may be evident—legal, marital, vocational, even medical—but cause and effect have become confused. The troubled nurse may attribute his or her irrational behavior and severe mood swings to an underlying emotional illness, rather than to the common effects of using mood-altering chemicals. The addict may perceive the alcohol or other drug merely as a pain reliever rather than as a source of addiction. The addict becomes entangled in a web of misapprehension and denial.

"Intervention" is the term used to describe a carefully planned, structured method of penetrating this web of denial and distorted perception. Through effective intervention, we help the chemically dependent nurse acknowledge the problem and present a believable solution. We stress that the goal of intervention is not to force a confession, but rather to elicit an agreement that the nurse will seek professional help for an evaluation of possible chemical dependency and treatment. Correctly transacted, intervention is highly successful.

The chemically dependent nurse acknowledges a problem, seeks professional evaluation, and pursues the recommended treatment. When this treatment is skilled and appropriate, the nurse can usually return to a healthy, productive professional and personal life.

KNOWING WHEN TO ACT

When a nurse is discovered "shooting up," stealing drugs, falsifying records, making blatant errors, or appearing at work acutely intoxicated, the need for action is clear. Most of the time, however, and especially early in the illness, the signs may not be obvious. Knowing when and how to respond is not so easy.

The symptoms of alcohol and other drug dependency are discussed in Chapter 2, as are the manifestations of denial in chemically dependent nurses and their co-workers, supervisors, friends, and family. Appropriate intervention begins with a willingness by those surrounding the troubled nurse to recognize and lower their defenses and confront difficult issues. Most people find it uncomfortable to consider a family member, friend, employee, or colleague chemically dependent. Even if we accept intellectually the reality of the disease, emotionally we may retain the stigma of addiction and hesitate to "accuse" a friend of a "denigrating" condition. It is important to understand this intellcctual–cmotional dichotomy. It is equally important to realize that it is not the role of friends and colleagues to diagnose chemical dependency. Rather, they must be aware of trouble signs—whatever the cause—and be prepared to respond appropriately.

Everyone has "bad days" and temporary troubles, but such episodes generally are limited. If a good-natured and competent colleague is moody or performs poorly, a friend or supervisor may ask what's wrong and offer to help. Ordinarily the troubled nurse will respond with explanations or apologies. The chemically dependent nurse is likely to respond to an expression of concern by denying the problem, blaming others, and rejecting help. Even if the chemically dependent person seems responsive, offers an explanation, and improves her behavior for a while, the problem *will* resurface, often with increasing frequency.

The supervisor faced with temporary or chronic problems should adhere to well-defined policies and procedures. Standard problem-solving methods should include objective documentation of unsatisfactory or deteriorating job performance, for the protection of the employee *and* the employer. If the nurse does not respond to usual problem-solving methods, intervention must be considered.

Case Study

The following adapted illustration is from *Professionals in Distress: Issues, Syndromes and Solutions in Psychology* (Kilburg, Nathan, & Thoreson, 1986, pp. 223–227). It is used with the permission of the American Psychological Association as well as R. Kilburg, P. Nathan, and R. Thoreson. We believe it demonstrates the distress experienced by all involved and the poor results when effective methods are not fully developed and implemented.

It is tempting to discuss only the successes, but a sense of what actually occurs during intervention attempts often promotes a richer understanding of the process, its problems, and the ultimate result of the intervention. The following case spanned five years.

> *Miss Jones was the clinical supervisor for a social work counseling service of a large public hospital. She was 61 years old, and had recurring mild back pain from a herniated disk. The problem could be managed without surgery through weight control, exercise, and correct posture. She had worked for the agency for approximately eight years, serving for the last two as supervisor of the off-site outpatient counseling and guidance service. She supervised a clinical staff of four social workers, one psychologist, and three counselors, all of whom were between 25 and 45 years old. Miss Jones had gradually become the agency's resident "alcohol expert" because she had attended a number of seminars and workshops on alcohol-related problems during the last five years.*

This last fact deserves a brief comment. We have noted with surprising regularity that when a clinical staff member in a "general service" community mental health clinic evolves into an alleged specialist in alcohol or drug abuse, the individual has often been self-selected because of personal problems in that area. Additionally, the agency may have urged that individual toward such a role in an indirect attempt to force him or her to confront an emerging problem. This indirect approach is rarely successful.

> *Some months after Miss Jones transferred to the off-site office, individual staff members noted an apparent deterioration in her work performance. She became less available for supervision of and consultation with staff members, less systematic in the review of cases, and erratic in keeping supervision appointments. She began to end supervision sessions abruptly after only 10 to 15 minutes. Moreover, clinical staff began to hear complaints from clients who had direct clinical contact with Miss Jones. Her administrative functioning appeared to be deteriorating; she seemed unable to produce necessary administrative reports, was erratic and inconsistent in administrative decision making, and was unable to follow through systematically on details.*
>
> *Concurrently, her co-workers noted other changes in personality and behavior. She appeared withdrawn and aloof. She spent less time chatting with staff and stopped sharing lunch hours with her co-workers. She was increasingly absent from work or would arrive at work late or leave early because "she was not feeling up to par." Clinical and clerical staff began to note alcohol on Miss Jones's breath during the afternoon and she appeared behaviorally "under the influence."*

Examination of all of the functional areas of a distressed professional often reveals a pattern that warrants concern and action. The casual observer probably would not notice small changes in an individual's behavior. A colleague who understood only one or two aspects of the individual's daily functions easily could perceive the less-than-effective performance as merely the result of a busy schedule, personal distraction, or similar "realistic" causes. At worst, a colleague might assess inappropriate individual behaviors as inadequate professional functioning or a mild example of poor professional judgment.

> *Initially, individual staff members privately commented to Miss Jones about various aspects of her behavior. Her response was defensive. She attributed her*

present difficulty to her "back problems," subtly suggested a lack of empathy on the part of the given staff member, and intimated that the staff member's "concern" was placing more pressure on her.

As the situation deteriorated and staff members' worries increased, they began to share their concerns with each other. They discovered that many of them had attempted individually to confront and support Miss Jones, without any apparent result. Finally, the clinical staff jointly confronted her about their observations—the administrative and clinical nonproductivity, the withdrawal from co-workers, and the evidence of drinking. She responded to the group as she had responded to them as individuals—she criticized them for not understanding, attacked them for making matters worse, and asking them to "back off" while she attended to her health problem. For a short time after the group confrontation, Miss Jones's functioning improved, but quickly resumed deterioration. Confronted a second time, her response was identical. After the second unsuccessful attempt, the staff decided to inform the hospital's program director about the situation.

The inability to successfully confront and support this individual was complicated by her intense and persistent denial, as well as by the public nature of the group confrontations during the latter stages of the attempted intervention. Furthermore, it is difficult, if not impossible, for subordinates in a work setting to successfully confront and assist their "boss," particularly when the confrontation occurs at the work site. Moreover, the "boss" is generally older than the subordinates and may consider them, because of their relative youth, personal and professional threats.

After receiving information about Miss Jones's behavior, the program director obtained collaborating evidence from clerical, administrative, and clinical staff. Despite Miss Jones's continued denials, countercharges, and explanations, the program director concluded that Miss Jones's functioning was not acceptable. She was given the choice of "doing something" to remedy the situation or indefinite leave, with a possibility of termination of em-

ployment. Miss Jones was told to work with an agency staff member who was the formally designated alcoholism treatment specialist and to report to that staff member on follow-through on an action plan.

The flaw in the administrative action is readily apparent. The program director, while firmly taking a stand in confronting the problem, established neither a clear and detailed plan for correcting the situation nor a clear set of procedures for approving and monitoring the plan or taking further administrative action. The staff member to whom Miss Jones was to report had no explicit authority to approve or disapprove her self-styled treatment plan. This type of ill-defined follow-up appears to be common. As we confront the distressed colleague, our guilt and doubt are too often manifest in our failing to develop a systematic and coherent set of expectations and require- ments. We unconsciously, or at least unintentionally, undermine our own attempt at confrontation as well as the likelihood of helping our colleague.

Miss Jones concluded that her drinking behavior was secondary to her health problem and that stress at work and in her personal life was a further "cause" of the drinking problem. Her self-developed plan to "do something" was to seek stress management counseling. The staff member responsible for monitoring the plan suggested that it was unlikely to ameliorate the situation, especially since the proposed stress management counseling was not going to focus on the alcohol use, and recommended that Miss Jones simultaneously attend Alcoholics Anonymous. Miss Jones rejected the suggestions, stating that she was in compliance with the agreement she made with the program director to "do something" by seeking the therapy of her choice. After a brief improvement, Miss Jones's performance, behavior, and drinking returned to their previous levels.

After the administrative staff found liquor bottles in her desk and filing cabinets, the program director placed her on indefinite administrative leave with the option that she seek undefined "appropriate help." If she adequately demonstrated a return to "normal functioning," she could return to her previous position. Miss Jones decided to seek voluntary hospitalization in a facility specializing in stress disorder treatment. While in the facility, she ultimately decided to seek early retirement for "health reasons."

This case highlights the extent of the denial process in chemical dependency. However, the most striking aspect of this case is the failure of ill-defined, nonspecific treatment and follow-up plans. By permitting Miss Jones to seek help from those without special expertise in alcoholism, her administrators almost guaranteed failure.

We like to believe that most problems can be handled within our usual systems, but the truth is that many of the modern attempts to deal with addictive illness remain barbaric.

INTERVENTION: FACING THE PROBLEM

Intervention tactics must be individualized and strategies may range from informal conversations with friends, to non-coercive peer assistance, to formal investigations and disciplinary actions. This discussion focuses on the formal, structured methods of intervention that may follow attempts at informal intervention and are most useful to family, friends, and employers.

Several intervention methods will be discussed. Each approach is based on the use of objective facts to confirm the dysfunction in the nurse's life, and each includes an element of surprise. The impaired nurse is not given in advance the reason for the initial meeting. While this "surprise element" may seem deceitful, it is a proven, effective method of overcoming denial, exposing concerns, and offering a means of friendly assistance. If forewarned, the nurse may either find an excuse not to participate, prepare a self-convincing, defensive rationalization, or manipulate the participants to the point of ineffectiveness. The elaborate defense system that develops with the illness will divert the usual attempts to discuss and solve an addiction problem. We also stress that intervention in chemical dependency must include a genuine concern and respect for the individual (King, 1986). The process is not a court of law aimed at convincing a jury or forcing a confession. There is no jury to convince; the "perpetrator" must be convinced and then treated. The intervenors are already aware of the problem. Their goal is to help, not to fire the employee or dismiss the problem and temporize until there is a tragedy.

The intervenors must have adequate training to perform their roles. Intervention must never be used as a means of punishment or a personal exercise of power. Its goal is to guide the chemically dependent nurse safely into treatment with as much gentleness as possible and only that degree of firmness and coercion required to attain the goal. It should not be attempted by the untrained, the half-trained, or the amateur.

If poorly handled, intervention can result in disaster. The chemically dependent person may feel unfairly attacked, rejected, even brutalized. The intervention technique, like a surgical instrument, is a powerful tool. Its value depends on the hands that wield it.

When intervention is properly conducted, the truth emerges and real concern is exhibited. Even if treatment is initially rejected, it may be accepted later. In any case, colleagues and friends will no longer deny the problem and their patterns of enabling the problem through "co-dependent" tolerance will be interrupted. There is almost always a long-range, positive effect for all concerned.

The Johnsonian Intervention

This popular method was developed by Vernon Johnson of the Johnson Institute in Minneapolis. It employs people who are meaningful in the chemically dependent person's life: a spouse, friends, children, colleagues, employers, parents, clergy, or anyone else with significant influence or importance. A professional in the addictions field usually prepares or trains this group, and is often present to facilitate the intervention, especially if the group members are new to the experience.

This approach, used in a family rather than a work setting, is described by Betty Ford (1987) in her recent autobiography. Her husband, children, a nurse, and a physician met in her home and shared their observations, their love and fear for her, and their sadness at her increasing distance as tranquilizers and alcohol pulled her away from them. Families of addicted nurses and the extended family of the workplace may not be identical, but the basic principles are similar.

The group meets in advance, considers and selects the objective information that will be presented, and carefully rehearses how the intervention will be conducted. They decide where and when the intervention will be held, the specific roles certain members of the group will play, the desired goal, and where the addicted person will receive follow-up evaluation or treatment. Each member must clearly understand what each participant will do if the evaluation is refused. Threats should not be made unless they can and will be acted upon. The professional guides the planning, recommends appropriate evaluation and treatment options, eliminates members who are too angry or excitable to avoid fighting and recrimination during the intervention, and serves as a facilitator. This type of intervention is used most often by groups with strong emotional ties to the chemically dependent person (V Johnson, 1986).

Peer Intervention

Peer intervention may include family members and other important people in the life of the chemically dependent person; however, it relies most on the influence of the person's professional peers. It is a colleague-to-colleague approach designed to motivate the person to agree to evaluation and treatment. As in other situations where the threat of job loss, real or implied, provides the coercive element, peers may use the threat of a report to the employer or the state board. The desired outcome—a decision to seek treatment—may be more predictable than when intervention is attempted only by family or neighbors with no serious consequences or threat to jobs if suggestions are refused.

These interventions are usually conducted by members of a peer assistance committee. Most often, this is a committee formed within the state nurses' association, although in some states it consists of a separate group of nurses. (Chapter 7 describes the various national structures.) The procedures may begin with a visit to the nurse by two volunteers. Ideally, one of the volunteers is a nurse in recovery from chemical dependency. The volunteers tell the nurse, without revealing the source, about the information that has come to their attention, and they ask for agreement to an evaluation. If necessary, they reveal the possible consequences (such as a report to the state board) of a refusal. They talk to the nurse about the disease of chemical dependency and the likelihood that the disease is the cause of the unprofessional, and perhaps, illegal behavior. The volunteers, stressing their desire to help, also offer the support and advocacy of the peer assistance program.

Depending on state laws and the peer assistance committee's policy, documentation of a peer intervention may not be extensive. The person who contacts the peer assistance committee is usually guaranteed anonymity, so that specific instances of inappropriate behavior are not available to the volunteers who first visit the nurse. To prevent vindictive use of the procedure, some committees require more than one verification of the behavior before they will take action. In these instances, however, confidential records of the callers are generally kept, indicating what was reported, the action taken, and the outcome. Note that in this situation, the nurse may be denied access to an accuser, but the action based on that accusation is still limited to an offer of help and is not a disciplinary action. If help is accepted at this point, no formal action may ever occur. The message, albeit unspoken, is that if early warnings are ignored, subsequent events may be more punitive. It is also implicit that what the nurse hoped and probably believed was a secret is no longer sacred.

Employment-Related Intervention

This type of intervention may be part of a formal hospital program such as an employee assistance program (EAP). It may be the informal work of an informed person or a group who realizes it is more beneficial to treat, rather than fire, chemically dependent employees (Bissell & Haberman, 1984; Sullivan, 1986). Many such people, former chemical dependents themselves, want to share their own positive experiences. This can be effective, but there are hazards in delegating too much responsibility to well-meaning but untrained and inexperienced people. A hospital clerk who was a recovered alcoholic developed a reputation as a problem solver for troubled employees. He was often asked by supervisors to counsel alcoholic employees, and was very effective with them. He was, however, driving them to a treatment facility in his own car, and risk-management concerns were raised concerning his quasi-official role as a hospital representative. Although the hospital continued to use his help, questions of process and documentation were brought under consideration.

Employment-related interventions always focus on evident job performance problems, including reduction in quantity or quality or work; problematic relationships with patients, co-workers or administrators; absenteeism; drug shortages; or combinations of these and other problems (see "Signs and Symptoms of Addiction," Chapter 2). Families are rarely involved in these interventions and the motivating factor is usually the threat of loss of position, a report to the state board of nursing, or both.

Documentation is very important. Records of previous attempts to rectify problems, indications of impairment, and job performance issues should be put in writing. It is important to remember that diagnosis of an illness is not required and is usually contraindicated in an intervention. The intervention is used to express concerns about the person and the work performance and to insist on an evaluation to establish the cause(s). Often addictive behaviors are associated with illnesses that can be treated successfully. Documentation of the intervention itself is also important. Record the participants, the material presented, the reaction of the nurse, the outcome, and the follow-up. A "confession" is unnecessary; rather, the goal is the nurse's agreement to submit to an evaluation. Agreements should be recorded very concisely, with no loopholes for future reinterpretation.

Combined Approaches

Intervention often requires a combination of the approaches described above. Co-workers or supervisors may be able to identify job impairment resulting from chemical dependency, but most hospitals do not have employee assistance programs. Hospital representatives are likely to contact a state nurses' association's peer assistance committee. These committees do not have the authority to conduct an investigation; however, once the committee identifies just cause, it may work with the hospital representative to plan the intervention. This is usually accomplished quickly, and the family is unlikely to be involved in the intervention. The motivating factor is the threat of further reporting, with job or license loss, and the alternative is evaluation and agreement to follow treatment recommendations. The preservation of employment is more likely to motivate the nurse to cooperate in the evaluation, follow the recommendations and bring job performance back to standards than will firing or threatening a report to the board. The peer assistance committee offers the impaired nurse the opportunity to participate in the peer assistance program, and stresses the availability of colleagues who care. This provides hope for recovery as well as a specific plan to enhance that recovery. The nurse will be monitored to ensure and verify continued recovery after treatment and resumption of work. The employer is assured that the program offers maximum protection to patients and to the institution, as well as help for the nurse. The documentation of post-treatment performance may seem unpleasant and invasive but many nurses have found it valuable. One nurse reported drugs stolen from her unit soon after she returned from treatment. Due to her history, she was the logical suspect. Because she had been closely monitored, she was able to prove that she had remained drug-free and the person who actually stole the drugs was identified.

The following example illustrates a combined approach. The setting is the hospital office of the director of nurses. The participants are aware of the facts and have prepared for the intervention. Narcotics counts have been frequently incorrect for several months. A recent incident involving one of the nurses resulted in a call to the peer assistance committee of the state nurses' association. The director of nurses (D.O.N) is present as are two members of the committee (MEM 1 and MEM 2), the subject's supervisor, (SUPER), and Barb, the subject of the concern. Barb has been summoned to the D.O.N.'s office. The D.O.N. begins the session.

D.O.N: Barb, I've called this meeting to discuss a very serious problem. I've invited these people to join us and you'll understand why in a minute. You'll have a chance to talk then. Do you agree? (*Barb nods agreement*) We've been concerned for a long time about narcotic counts on your unit. On Tuesday, it was reported that you were seen placing syringes in your purse before you went home. Later that shift, patients said they were not getting relief from their pain medication. When we checked, we discovered their medications had been replaced with sterile water.

BARB: Now wait a minute! (*Getting angry, leans forward in her chair*) What do you think you're accusing me of!?

D.O.N.: I asked you to wait until we were finished, Barb, and you agreed. You'll have an opportunity to talk.

(*Barb sits back, obviously still unhappy*)

SUPER: We've also been concerned for some time about the change in you, Barb. You're one of our best nurses and everybody likes you, but lately there have been times when you're very hard to get along with. You're moody; people are afraid you're going to jump down their throats and sometimes you do. There are days when you even look awful, as though you're sick.

D.O.N: Something's going on, Barb, and we want you to be evaluated and find out what it is.

BARB: Is that all you want? I'll go see Dr. Jones this afternoon.

D.O.N: Dr. Jones won't do, Barb. We want you to be evaluated by a chemical dependency professional as part of the state nurses' association peer assistance program.

BARB: You think I'm a drug addict! I'm not going to let you get away with this! I won't agree, I'm going to see a lawyer.

MEM 1: Barb, if you want to see a lawyer, you certainly should, but let me explain to you how we can help. *(Explains the program to her)*

MEM 2: Barb, I want to tell you a little about my own experience. Over two years ago, I was in the same spot you're in. I didn't want to admit it, but I had known for a long time that I couldn't stop on my own. I was given the same chance you're getting now. I took off work for two months, and I've been straight now for almost two years. Barb, it feels so good, it's such a relief! This program can help you just like it helped me.

BARB: *(To the D.O.N.)* What about my job? *(Tears are forming in her eyes)*

D.O.N: If you follow the treatment recommendations, stay in the program, and do your part, you'll keep your job and we won't have to report this to the board. If you don't agree, though, Barb, we have no choice but to let you go and to call the board.

BARB: *(Looks at the floor, tears falling, and speaks softly)* I'll co-operate. I knew this would happen. My God, I'm glad it's over!

Documentation of the content of any employment-related intervention is essential. Depending on state law and peer assistance committee policy, documentation may be the responsibility of the hospital representative or may be augmented by the committee. It is often useful to prepare a document of agreement for the nurse and the major participants to sign or initial immediately. This will help prevent future reinterpretations or misunderstandings.

The Well-Planned Intervention

During intervention preparation, each participant should understand exactly what is expected, including the material each is responsible for presenting. Here are some helpful guidelines (Jefferson & Ensor, 1982):

1. Conduct the intervention while the events are fresh; time dampens motivation, obscures detail, and alters memory.

2. Prepare written documentation of each participant's concerns; address direct observations. Include notes on specific times, dates, and witnesses.

3. State the desired outcome and the consequences if it is not reached. (Do not accept the nurse's vague promises to improve performance or quit drug use without outside help; most chemically dependent people are very adept at rationalization and manipulation.) Anticipate the nurse's likely objections to entering treatment (such as lack of child care, previous commitments, need to discuss things with family, or financial limitations) and make advance plans to counter them. Scheduling the necessary time to get well *will* disrupt routines and even vacation plans.

4. Present the material in a kind and caring manner, but be firm. Moral outrage, anger, or sympathy may contribute to the problem.

5. Be prepared to follow through after the intervention. Enlist a staff member to accompany the nurse to a treatment center immediately, if necessary. Do not permit an intoxicated person to drive. Do not postpone the next action. The evaluation should take place without delay. The intervenors should be alert to the possibility that the nurse may be suicidal. If the nurse does not agree to immediate evaluation, family members or close friends should be informed of what has occurred and warned to take whatever precautions are necessary.

6. Create a record as soon as the intervention is complete.

Intervention participants are frequently concerned that the nurse will become very angry, walk out of the meeting, and remain angry. This is rare. Most often the nurse will react like Barb, above. He or she will listen and may act defensive but will rarely become aggressive. More often the nurse will express relief that the ordeal of concealment is over.

When the nurse agrees to an evaluation, participants experience a sense of relief. It may be tempting to end the intervention at this point. The next steps, however, are also important. The nurse should be expected to:

1. Follow the recommendations resulting from the evaluation, which will likely include extended treatment.

2. Cooperate with the peer assistance program and/or Employee Assistance Program (EAP).

3. Improve and maintain work performance at an acceptable level.

If the nurse does not agree to the evaluation, the intervention participants must stress that they will act immediately on what they have presented as consequences for such a decision. If the nurse does not follow the treatment recommendations or drops out of treatment the same consequences will apply. This follow-up motivates the nurse to accept the initial recommendation and enter treatment. It also protects the patients under the nurse's care, and it preserves the integrity of the peer assistance approach and the profession. Expectations must be clear; agreements must be honored meticulously. If promises, positive or negative, are kept, mutual trust and respect will prevail.

Nursing, like other professions, has its grapevine. Colleagues will eventually hear stories of addiction. A recovering nurse may even tell the story herself. If a supervisor or hospital committee has a reputation for being supportive or helpful, colleagues will be more likely to report each other, rather than feeling they must protect their friends from a supervisor's indignation, outrage, or perhaps even vengeance.

When properly conducted, intervention is a highly successful method of addressing a difficult problem. The prospect of conducting an intervention may be frightening. Intervenors with many years of practice in successful interventions will admit to dry throats, racing pulses, and searches for last-minute escape hatches. It will, indeed, often be unpleasant, even painful. It is, however, a preferable alternative to firing, which usually leaves one with a sense of failure or loss. A successful intervention may save a career, a family, even a life.

CHAPTER 4

TREATMENT

There are more chemical dependency treatment resources available today than at any other time in history. Programs differ in technique, client focus, and, unfortunately, quality. Effective treatment programs include the family in the treatment process and have two basic goals for all their patients: Abstinence from all mood-altering drugs of addiction and ongoing participation in an appropriate 12-step program.

These two conditions, we believe, are universally necessary for a complete and sustained recovery. Because chemical dependency is a chronic illness, recovery is not merely attained but must be maintained with diligence.

Even if other physical and/or psychological disorders are present, the chemical dependency must be recognized as a primary disease and treated accordingly. Additional illnesses and life situations must also be considered. Effective treatment will be flexible and individualized.

INDIVIDUALIZING TREATMENT

The nursing model of self-care is often effective in chemical dependency treatment. Orem (1985) suggests that patients need nurs-

care only when they cannot care for themselves. With this approach, treatment actively done "for" and "to" the patient is in inverse relation to the patient's realistic ability to care for him/herself. The self-care model is appropriate for work with chemically dependent patients (Bennett, Vourakis, & Woolf, 1983). Graves (1982) also takes into consideration the strong denial system and resulting incapacity to determine "realistic ability" for self-care. The concept of self-care may be helpful in determining an appropriate course of treatment, with the caveat that the chemically dependent person may not be able to assess realistically what can be accomplished. A variety of factors must be considered in determining the optimum approach for each individual.

Physiologic Factors and Nature of the Addiction

Alcohol is a toxic drug, and even short-term use can have long-term effects that become more severe over time. Although the amount of alcohol consumed is not the determining factor in diagnosing alcoholism, alcoholics usually do consume large quantities of the drug.

The acute effects of alcohol range from simple drunkenness to severe central nervous system depression, respiratory arrest, and death. The long-range effects of chronic alcohol use may include severe damage to many body systems.

Sedative–hypnotic drugs, including barbiturates, chloral hydrate, benzodiazepines, and others, also have toxic and long-term effects. Most of these drugs have the ability to depress the central nervous system to the point of death. Alcohol used in combination with these drugs may enhance their action. The half-life of such drugs varies from three hours to well over a hundred hours, during which time the drug or metabolite may be active in the body.

Toxic levels of central nervous system stimulants such as amphetamines and cocaine produce overstimulated systems, resulting in paranoia, delusion, hallucinations, seizures, blood pressure and heart rate elevation, vomiting, and diarrhea. Death may result from cardiac arrest, arrythmia, hyperthermia, or stroke.

Narcotics are part of a group of drugs known as opioids, also known as analgesics. They can produce mood changes, drowsiness, and respiratory distress. Long-term effects include gastrointestinal involvement sometimes resulting in obstruction. Although cocaine is not actually a narcotic, it is a controlled substance and is therefore included in narcotics legislation.

Tolerance (the ability of the body to handle increasing amounts of a drug) develops with prolonged use of most of these drugs. There may be no noticeable signs of intoxication, however, there may be physical complications that reflect the method of use, such as deterioration of the nasal septum due to long-term snorting of cocaine, "track marks" over veins, or infections due to careless techniques or the sharing of needles. For the pregnant addict, there may be damage to the fetus since many drugs cross the placental barrier.

The physical effects, illnesses, and complications secondary to chemical dependency are boundless. There are even certain cancers associated with chemical dependency. A thorough physical examination to determine the health status of the nurse should always be conducted early in the treatment process.

The Patient's Attitude and Motivation

We have already discussed the role of denial in the disease of chemical dependency. The addict commonly underestimates the difficulty in achieving a solid recovery and will bargain to invest as little effort as possible in treatment. A first response is often, "I'll do it myself." Excuses, like "I need to care for my children" or "I'm not a group person," may be offered as resistance to intensive treatment. The addict may offer to take Antabuse®, a drug that produces nausea, vomiting, flushing, sweating, and faintness if drinking occurs, or Trexan®, a drug that blocks the effects of opiates.

Such equivocation about a long-term treatment program is not a sign of poor motivation or ill will. It is part of the process of recognizing and accepting the need for treatment. This illness distorts the patient's perceptions of reality, and the treatment plan must be the result of informed, clear thinking. This is not the time to negotiate. For example, the nurse who is well-groomed, articulate, and thus far has retained the respect of peers may try to convince the intervenor that inpatient treatment is unnecessary, when in fact the extent and strength of the denial may necessitate an inpatient experience to penetrate the defense system.

The following example of an inadequate treatment plan conceived after negotiation with the patient involved a nurse who had been using 30 ccs of Demerol® daily for two years. A disciplinary body agreed to weekly outpatient treatment by a mental health professional with no specialized training in addiction. The therapist made an attempt to learn why the nurse was using Demerol and then prescribed tranquilizers. No specific effort was focused on helping the nurse control her addiction. When she proved "uncooperative" by continuing to take the drugs, her license was revoked.

The choice of treatment cannot be left entirely to the addicted nurse. Treatment of chemical dependency cannot be done at the nurse's convenience and personal comfort should not be a determining factor in selecting the appropriate approach.

The Nurse as Patient

There is much debate on the appropriate treatment setting for nurses and other professionals. Should nurses be treated in settings designed especially for health care professionals, or can they be successfully treated among people with a variety of backgrounds? Little data are available to substantiate arguments for either approach (Bissell & Haberman, 1984). Experience shows, however, that a variety of treatment programs have been successfully treating nurses and others for a number of years. It is more important that chemically dependent nurses participate in high-quality programs in facilities that understand nurses' unique problems with addiction and recovery. Therapists must be familiar with the professional and regulatory environment to which recovering nurses will return.

The addicted nurse may have difficulty assuming the role of patient (Bennett, Vourakis, & Woolf, 1983). Personal anecdotes are plentiful, such as the hospitalized nurse who changed the linens on her own bed or the one who made it her responsibility to care for her roommate. The nurse in treatment must be encouraged temporarily to relinquish the role of caretaker (Jaffe, 1982).

A chemically dependent nurse in treatment may have to cope with extreme feelings of guilt due to incompetent behavior on the job, particularly if patients were endangered or harmed. Nurses may be more likely than other women in treatment to feel humiliation and shame, since the expectation, as with other health professionals, is that a nurse "should know better." While few nurses entering treatment report that their drug use resulted in patient suffering or physical harm, they nevertheless very feel guilty about their situation (Bissell & Haberman, 1984; Jaffe, 1982). We have heard many times, "I can't be alcoholic, I'm a nurse."

Because of their education, nurses frequently attempt to intellectualize their illnesses, reading the current literature and becoming very clinical and objective. This curiousity is not necessarily a drawback, since it provides the nurse with solid information about chemical dependency rather than the assumptions and misinformation that often abound. It is important, however, that the emotional aspects are addressed during the treatment process. The nurse cannot be allowed to trade the patient role for that of expert in an attempt to continue denial, assume control, and avoid treatment.

It is essential that the treatment program staff have an understanding of the dynamics of nursing and the effects of culture and practice of the profession on the nurse's recovery and acceptance of the patient role during treatment. One nurse was referred to a treatment program after diverting drugs from her work setting during a period of 18 months. There was a bartender in treatment with her, who was told during group therapy that he should find another job, since being around alcohol would likely cause a relapse. The nurse was told, in the same session, that she should get back to work in nursing as soon as she finished the inpatient program. This recommendation demonstrated little understanding of the effect of proximity of the drug of choice for this nurse.

Since there are indications that the nursing profession attracts people who are children of alcoholics, the chemically dependent nurse in treatment may also have co-dependency treatment needs. Commonly reported symptoms of co-dependency (Cermak, 1986; Wegscheider, 1983) are:

○ Self-esteem that relies heavily on feeling needed by others

○ Attempts to control others even when it is unrealistic to do so

○ Development of complicated relationships with chemically dependent people

These symptoms could easily contribute to or cause relapse if not considered during evaluation and treatment.

Other Factors

Each nurse's personal life and background will require special evaluation during the treatment process. Gender is also an important factor. Many female nurses in treatment for chemical dependency report that their identity as women and the problems they face as women were more important considerations in the treatment process than what they happened to do for a living. The self-esteem of women in treatment is often described as lower than that of men in treatment. Women are more likely to report feeling anxious and depressed, and suicide attempts are more common. In addition, the divorce rate of women in recovery from chemical dependency is higher than for men, and, if they have children, they often perceive themselves as poor parents, for which they feel guilt (Bissell & Haberman, 1984; Blume, 1986). The guilt is likely to be particularly strong if they have abused or neglected a child, or if the child was affected *in utero* by chemicals used during pregnancy. Even the prolonged absence required for inpatient treatment may be perceived as further abandoning family responsibilities.

Male nurses may have the "advantage" that most treatment centers, halfway houses, clinics, and diagnostic tests have been planned for men and standardized accordingly. However, male nurses represent a tiny minority of their profession, and thus a nurse-oriented treatment program may not be as sensitive to unique factors in a man's life.

Sexual orientation may also be an important factor in selection of a treatment program. Because acceptance of homosexuality is not universal, the gay or lesbian nurse should receive treatment where the caregivers are sensitive to their sexual orientation. Although people's secrets may isolate them and interfere with recovery, candor in the wrong setting could ruin a career. Today, the added fear of AIDS ostracizes homosexuals even more. Thus assurance of discretion is vital in choosing treatment.

Religious background presents important considerations as well. For instance, staff may be unaware of important dietary laws or spiritual issues. The traditional AA program is a Christian approach; Jews in treatment often have been expected to take a "fifth step" with a Catholic priest.[1] At one treatment facility, staff did not understand

---

[1]The fifth step is an action suggested but not required by AA in which a member shares candidly with one other trusted person both alcoholism history and present situation. It is not catharsis or confession in the usual sense but does contain elements of both; it is a moral housecleaning.

why an orthodox Jewish man needed prayer time each morning or why he resisted clasping hands with a woman patient while intoning the Lord's Prayer at the end of a group meeting.

Ethnicity is another important factor requiring special sensitivity. Racism and xenophobia (excessive fear and hatred of those different from oneself, especially foreigners) do exist among patients and staff of treatment programs, and this factor cannot be ignored however un-pleasant it is. There are specialized treatment facilities for some minority groups, although these may not be well designed for women or sensitive to the special problems of nurses. American Indian, black, and Latino AA groups tend to be strongly male-oriented. There are only a handful of residential treatment programs with staff fluent in Spanish or other non-English languages. Few understand Asian cultures.

Other personal factors which must be considered are family situation, proximity of the treatment site to family and friends, age, and any other special situation important in the life of the individual.

It is usually impossible to find a setting that addresses all the above considerations. Unfortunately some institutions and state nursing association peer assistance programs for impaired professionals establish contractual relationships with only one or a few treatment facilities. With such limited choices available, some individuals with special needs will be disappointed. Wherever possible, a variety of resources and an expert referral counselor should be available to ensure that selection of a treatment program is made with the interest of the patient in mind.

The Continuum of Care

Recovery from chemical dependency occurs along a continuum, progressing from the intensive stages of withdrawal and primary care, through a program of continuing treatment, to an indefinite period of "self-care."

Withdrawal

When a nurse becomes physically dependent on alcohol or other drugs there follows a period of physical withdrawal as the alcohol or drugs are discontinued. The severity and nature of the withdrawal is determined by the nature of the drug(s) used, the amount and duration of use, the presence of other physical problems, and the physiological and psychological response of the individual user. The withdrawal period (detoxification) is often handled on an inpatient basis, but some patients may be able to manage this phase on an outpatient basis, depending on the drug involved (some drugs do not produce physical withdrawal symptoms), the length and degree of addiction, and the outcomes of any previous attempts to stop drug use. The degree of organic damage, particularly to the central nervous system, must also be considered. Withdrawal can be so subtle and mild that the addict may not notice it. Measurable pupillary dilitation during propoxyphine (Darvon®) withdrawal, for instance, may not be apparent to the addict.

The withdrawal experience varies widely among chemically dependent people. It even varies for the same person from episode to episode, although a patient's history of previous episodes is generally accepted to be a good predictor of the course of current withdrawal. The caretakers' ability to offer real hope and reassurance of lasting recovery will affect the withdrawal experience and assist the patient in overcoming the withdrawal symptoms and diminish depression and suicide risks. There are still nurses who have had little or no experience with current withdrawal practices. Their own experience may have been with undermedicated alcoholic patients who were hallucinating, in restraints, and obviously miserable. The nurse may be unaware that delerium tremens, seizures, and most of the painful and dangerous symptoms of the withdrawal state are generally preventable. In skilled hands, the patient in withdrawal faces little physical discomfort. A nurse who is still able to function minimally can, even if taking enormous quantities of alcohol and other drugs, anticipate remaining under close observation but ambulatory and free of IVs. All that will be required of the nurse is candor about the type and quantity of drugs recently used.

Cocaine and amphetamines, although highly addictive, show relatively mild physical withdrawal signs but can produce severe depression, anhedonia, subjective discomfort, and drug hunger. Grand mal seizures are common in abrupt and untreated alcohol withdrawal just as they can appear as toxic manifestations of excessive injection of cocaine and narcotics.

Some withdrawal situations require medication and sophisticated hospital treatment, others need only time. It is a common mistake to identify withdrawal as only that period during which a drug is leaving the body and to assume that once the drug is entirely absent the process is complete.

Actually, many drugs disappear quite rapidly. If alcohol is used alone, it is usually gone within 24 hours after the last drink. There may be after-effects, however. If heavy drinking occurs on a single evening, withdrawal poses little danger, although there may be an unpleasant hangover the morning after. (Note that driving ability and other skills will be impaired during the hangover period.) If drinking has been heavy for a prolonged period, withdrawal symptoms may range from mild to severe. There may be tachycardia, fever, increased blood pressure, and slight-to-gross intention tremor. With greater physical addiction there may be grand mal seizures (referred to in the past as "rum fits"), auditory, tactile, or visual hallucinations, and disorientation. The severe form of withdrawal, with tremors and disorientation, is referred to as the D.T.s (delerium tremens, the "shaking delerium"). Untreated or ineptly treated, severe D.T.s can end in death.

Withdrawal from other sedative, hypnotic drugs including the "minor" tranquilizers can result in a form of D.T.s, although the severity and time sequence of withdrawal events will differ for each drug. Librium® and Valium® are excreted very slowly—they are usually not fully cleared from the body for about a week—so the withdrawal period is more prolonged.

Physical dependency on alcohol and other sedatives can cause a more significant physical addiction and withdrawal state than opiates. Alcohol and barbiturate withdrawal can result in death. Narcotic withdrawal can be miserable but is rarely fatal. Opiate use generates more controversy because of its illegal status, the fact that it is often injected rather than swallowed, and because of the regulations and procedures associated with its controlled status. Compared to alcohol withdrawal, the primary physical complications from opiate withdrawal are much less serious.

Withdrawal treatment follows the same pattern and approach for both sedatives and opiates. If drugs are required, a long-acting substitute for the drug of addiction is given in decreasing amounts over a short period of time, so that the patient is gradually tapered off the drug rather than suddenly deprived of it. Paraldehyde, associated with unexplained sudden deaths, is rarely used since other and better drugs are available. The phenothiazines are also avoided because they increase risk of convulsions. Phenytoin (Dilantin®) will not prevent seizures caused by withdrawal. The most common drugs used to treat withdrawal are phenobarbital or benzodiazapine, usually Librium or Valium. Methadone is still used for opiate withdrawal in some programs; clonidine, a newer non-addicting drug, is used increasingly.

Withdrawal regimens vary from one "detox" unit or treatment center to another but the basic principles remain the same. The goal also remains the same: To free the patient from all addictive drugs as safely, comfortably, and quickly as possible. The use of amino acids is popular, along with certain tricyclic antidepressants, in treatment of cocaine withdrawal.

There are also mental and emotional aspects to withdrawal; however, it may be difficult to ascertain what is due to toxicity, what is a natural part of the withdrawal state, and what is permanent brain damage. During alcohol and other sedative withdrawal, agitation and depression are common, but in most cases disappear rapidly. Problems with recent memory, and inability to concentrate and abstract are also frequently reported. Many recovered addicts report that they felt effects for as much as a year after the last drug and they were aware of the severity of their addiction only in retrospect. This does not imply that they were unable to function or safely return to work. Healing takes time and there may be joyless periods of "Is this all there is?" One nurse who followed a close friend through the first year of recovery said, "Although she seemed perfectly fine, I really saw the difference at the end of a year when the sparkle returned to her eyes."

In most settings, medication of some type is used to prevent or diminish the discomfort experienced during detoxification. The better treatment centers administer this kind of medication carefully to avoid conveying the unspoken message that a drug is the answer to all discomfort, and to keep the patient alert enough to interact with others during the detoxification process.

Some withdrawal programs, known as social-setting detoxification programs, rely on the interaction and relationship between staff and the patient population to minimize withdrawal symptoms. These treatment centers are not in hospitals: Most are private group homes or dormitory settings. Many are insistently "non-medical" and, although they do take vital signs, will not dispense drugs. They provide a structured and drug-free environment in which people can withdraw with the same physical and social care they might get from a supportive friend. The group leader is often a nurse. If an addict appears physically ill, he or she is taken to a hospital for evaluation and treatment. This is a successful form of withdrawal; only about 5% of all patients admitted to such programs have required transfer to a medical facility for medication (O'Briant & Lennard, 1973).

Detoxification that requires medication is usually managed on an inpatient basis. While some physicians do prescribe drugs on a temporary outpatient basis, this is generally not recommended because of the potential for abuse of the prescribed drug. Under no circumstances should more medication be given to the patient than would be safe if the patient were to take it all at once or in combination with alcohol or another drug.

The home environment may also pose danger during withdrawal. If the patient returns to an angry or punitive spouse, lives with another addict or alcoholic, or faces a stressful home or work situation, the atmosphere is unlikely to provide enough support through a difficult withdrawal process. Daily visits with knowledgeable treatment personnel are recommended if outpatient detoxification is attempted.

Primary Care

After the withdrawal process has cleared the drug from the physiologic system the intensive initial treatment known as *primary care* may begin. The successful primary treatment programs include a combination of therapy and education. Therapy focuses on management of the acute problems—physical, psychological, social, or spiritual—that have resulted from the disease. Whenever possible, the family, extended family, or significant others are included in the therapy process. A family develops debilitating symptoms while living with a chemical dependent. The nature of the symptoms should be identified and addressed, with plans made and initial steps taken toward addressing these symptoms.

Understanding one's disease is as important in the treatment of chemical dependency as it is in the treatment of other chronic illnesses. Patients and their families must learn about the illness for the same reasons that diabetic or cardiovascular patients must learn about theirs. In addition, there are many myths and negative attitudes to overcome. If health professionals are uninformed and naive about chemical dependency, so, too, is the addict, who may have collected misinformation to justify continued use.

A combination of group and individual therapy is the most common approach to treatment. Both forms of therapy should encourage each patient to internalize the concepts that are presented in the educational portion of the program. Therapy will also address other issues, some of which may be held in common with other patients. Many patients are initially reluctant to participate in group therapy. Group therapy is important, however, because the group process accomplishes several things:

1. It allows patients to share commonalities and dissipates their feeling of uniqueness.

2. It confronts the remaining denial and rationalizations in a powerful manner.

3. It offers positive support for healthy coping behaviors.

4. It allows the patient to help other group members.

Individual therapy should also be part of treatment. Regardless of the closeness and effectiveness of the group, not all patients will be able to express their concerns during the three or four weeks of inpatient treatment.

Primary care may occur in either inpatient or outpatient settings. Inpatient treatment, whether at a hospital or a freestanding facility, generally lasts 21 to 28 days although exceptions do occur and should not necessarily be interpreted as excessive. Outpatient care consists of two basic approaches: (a) the traditional program, in which the patient participates in individual, family, or group therapy for one or two hours per week for an indeterminate period of time, or (b) the more recently introduced intensive outpatient treatment, in which the patient and often family members attend sessions for several hours at a time, two to five times a week for four to eight weeks. These intensive treatment programs are sometimes called "day hospital," "night hospital," "partial hospitalization," or "day program." Some intensive outpatient programs operate predominantly on weekends and evenings to allow patients to continue full-time work. Others demand a full-time commitment: The patient attends an inpatient program during the day but sleeps at home. Research (Blume, 1986) has shown little variance in the success rates of inpatient versus outpatient treatment programs.

Continuing Care

The continuing care period is sometimes referred to as "aftercare." We have deliberately avoided the use of that term because we believe it is not an "extra" or a less important phase that follows the "real" treatment. Primary treatment is only the beginning of the recovery process. In fact, some therapists consider primary treatment preparation for the true treatment of the illness, which occurs during continuing care. Recovery does not occur spontaneously when alcohol or other drug use ceases.

After completion of primary treatment, continuing treatment can be expected for at least a year—and perhaps two or three years—depending on the needs of individual patients and their families (Royce, 1981). Continuing therapy may consist of group, individual, family therapy, or a combination. Some patients require a period of additional support in a halfway house or transitional residence. With this method, the nurse can reenter the workplace while receiving the benefits of therapy and support.

During the continuing care period, complicating factors such as learning parenting skills, settling old issues of an abusive parent, doing long-range career planning, working through long-standing sexual problems, or other psychological or emotional issues may be addressed. Physiologic problems are considered as well. Many physical problems like mild adult-onset diabetes, idiopathic grand mal seizures, mild essential hypertension, and even anxiety and depression will vanish as the addiction is treated.

Self-Care

Primary treatment should always include education about and exposure to Alcoholics Anonymous, Cocaine Anonymous, and/or Narcotics Anonymous and the corresponding groups for family members, Al-Anon and Nar-Anon. These groups do not describe themselves as "treatment providers"; each describes itself as a fellowship. They provide a 12-step structured recovery program and an arena for sharing experience, strength, and hope. The only requirement for membership is a desire to stop drinking/using. Anyone interested in the field of chemical dependency is encouraged to attend open meetings and study the literature of these groups.

It is important to note that the formation of Alcoholics Anonymous in 1935 preceded by 20 years the formal redesignation of alcoholism as a disease by most health care groups. Despite its status as a disease, alcoholism was originally termed "inebriety." During Prohibition, alcoholism was considered a sin rather than illness, an attitude that has required conscious effort to reverse. The modern field of chemical dependency treatment was spawned by AA. Many people working in the field today are members of Alcoholics Anonymous, Narcotics Anonymous, or Al-Anon, which accounts for the strong sense of "we" between patients and staff. Those accustomed to a more traditional differentiation between patients and staff may be uncomfortable with this group attitude. The specific role of these support groups to nurses is discussed more completely in Chapter 6.

After the extended period of continuing care, indefinite—usually lifelong—participation in mutual help groups is generally considered necessary for sustained recovery. The prototypical mutual support group is Alcoholics Anonymous. The founder of AA called himself a stockbroker, although he actually was not. According to his wife, Lois, he completed law school but failed one fourth year course, so technically never graduated and was not, therefore, a professional. The second member was a physician, the third an attorney, and one of the earliest women members was a nurse. Groups have formed recently to address other addictive illnesses. Narcotics Anonymous (NA) and Cocaine Anonymous (CA) help those addicted to narcotics, while Overeaters Anonymous (OA) applies the AA principles to compulsive eating disorders. Similar groups founded to help people live with diseases, disorders, or general life problems include Pills Anonymous, Drugs Anonymous, Emotions Anonymous (for emotional dysfunction) Make Today Count (for cancer patients), Candlelighters (for parents of deceased children), and Recovery (for former psychiatric patients). There are within AA many special interest groups, such as those speaking a common foreign language. There are AA groups conducted in sign language. In New York there is a group for people with AIDS. Women's groups and youth groups are widely available. Addresses of the national offices of the major mutual help/resource organizations are listed in Appendix E.

The principles of AA, and of many similar mutual-help groups, are simple. They are based on the assumption that the condition is not controlled at one's will and addictive behavior cannot be quelled by mere exertion of extra efforts. Therefore, the addict must give up control to a "higher power," which can be anything *outside* of the person (a god, treatment center, or AA group). AA commonly refrains, "You don't have to believe in God so long as you know it's not you" and "Together we can do what no one of us can do in isolation." It is a paradox of recovery that when a person relinquishes control, the dependency condition becomes controllable; that is, it is no longer an insurmountable obstacle (Brown, 1985). There have been many attempts to explain the mechanism of the AA philosophy (Glaser & Ogborne, 1982; Kurtz, 1982; Maxwell, 1962, 1984) but these theoretical explanations are of little concern to its members. Many people who tried very hard for years to control their drinking or other drug use and regularly failed credit AA for relief of their distress.

Membership in AA or NA is open to anyone with the desire to stop drinking or taking other drugs. One joins by deciding he or she *is* a member. There are no dues or fees, and only informal membership records (if any) are kept. The groups are autonomous and each group has a representative on a local board of governors. This board serves primarily to disseminate information to the groups. The groups are run by members and employ a consensus decision-making mechanism know as the "group conscience" in which each member searches his/ her conscience and agrees on the decision. Each group decides the topics of discussion, as well as the time and place of meetings. Each AA member may attend as many or as few weekly meetings as he or she wishes, however, one meeting a week is designated a "home group." Regular weekly attendance at that meeting is common, but still not required.

An AA practice known as sponsorship provides additional support to members. They may select a "sponsor," who agrees to assist with recovery by providing individualized direction, pointing out potential consequences of planned action, and acting as a more personalized resource for the AA program. Sponsors are usually chosen from among the more experienced members who have a longer period of sobriety than the requesting member. Relationships between sponsor and member vary considerably, with some pairs developing friendships and others limiting their relationship to matters related to the member's recovery.

There are mutual-help groups for family members of chemical dependents and co-dependents. Al-Anon, an offshoot of AA, is for children, spouses, parents, and friends of alcoholics and Alateen is available for teenage children of alcoholics. Adult Children of Alcoholics groups are also prevalent. A description of co-dependency treatment is beyond the scope of this text but resources are listed in the Selected References following the text.

NURSES' SUPPORT GROUPS

When nurses join AA, they may experience unique problems. Many members of AA have used alcohol exclusively or in combination with other oral drugs (very often legal prescriptions) or marijuana. Nurses may have used injectable narcotics obtained from patients or stolen from the hospital. In addition, they probably cared for patients while they were "under the influence." Other AA members may reflect society's abhorrence for drug addicts or be shocked by the drug-taking nurse. Acceptance and the identification of similar experiences is vitally important when the nurse begins the difficult road to sustained recovery. Rejection rather than support from one's group could seriously imperil recovery. Recovering nurses often say that they cannot talk freely about their drug use in an AA meeting. There may be fear of lawsuits if a member of the group should prove untrustworthy when the nurse admits to caring for patients while actively using or drinking. A nurse may choose Narcotics Anonymous, but many NA members are former "street addicts," so the nurse may feel unable to share experiences there either. Some nurses attend both AA *and* NA.

Support groups for nurses have been formed to address the specific problems of nurses in recovery. The groups may be initiated by treatment centers to help their former patients, by the local nurses' association, by a private counselor, or by a group of recovering nurses. A few groups contain a variety of health care professionals. In these groups, many of which are modeled after AA, nurses feel more free to discuss their experiences as well as their feeling of shame and guilt about violating their own ethical principles, especially if they have been stealing or jeopardizing patients. Members who have successfully resolved these issues share their strength and hope with newer members. These groups, however, are not a substitute for primary AA or NA meetings. They supplement but do not replace them. Nurses' support groups will be discussed further in Chapter 6.

ASSESSING THE QUALITY OF A TREATMENT PROGRAM

Unfortunately, not all treatment programs are equal in quality. Most programs are staffed by health care professionals (physicians, nurses, social workers, psychologists, and counselors). However, the basic educational preparation for these professions does not always foster the knowledge and skills necessary to work effectively with the chemical dependent. This expertise is generally acquired through continuing education programs, workshops, and seminars in the diagnosis and treatment of chemical dependency.[2]   Thus it is important to investigate the staff's credentials in the field of chemical dependency.

To avoid pitfalls in treatment, look for a multidisciplinary team approach that specializes in chemical dependency treatment and has a demonstrable track record of success. The least desirable choice would be an individual with a generic mental health background operating as a private entrepreneur with few, if any, colleagues. A recovered nurse who has experienced chemical dependency may offer a special dimension in role modeling, understanding, and identification, however. Many alcoholics and addicts attempt treatment of other doctors or nurses when they have been sober for only brief periods themselves. They may have little more than enthusiasm or zealotry to offer, in addition to inadequate training and preparation. Some become interested in the role because of a family member's addiction, which may now be resolved and genuinely useful as background; others are still in turmoil. Some enthusiasts are still actively and harmfully involved with alcohol or other drugs but are in denial and still not suspected by peers.

An important credential in this field is that of Certified Alcoholism and/or Drug Addiction Counselor (the specific title may vary from state to state). This competency-based credential requires that the bearer meet specifically defined criteria in the treatment of alcohol

---

[2]There are a few university- and college-based programs in addictions, but they vary in quality, and are not extensive enough to produce large numbers of trained staff.

and/or other drug addicts. While the educational background of people with this credential may range from a high school diploma to a PhD, they will all have specific education in chemical dependency and have practiced in the field under supervision for a specified time. Efforts are currently under way to standardize these criteria nationally.

Other recent developments in credentialing include a new credential for the Employee Assistance Program Counselor provided by ALMACA (Association of Labor Management Administrators and Consultants in Alcoholism), and a physicians' credential offered under the auspices of the American Medical Society on Alcoholism and Other Drugs of Dependency (AMSAODD). The first written examination for this credential was conducted in 1986. In addition, the National Nurses Society on Addictions (NNSA) is currently working with the American Nurses' Association (ANA) to develop a certification for nurses. The Joint Commission on the Accreditation of Hospitals has accredited specialized programs, but the accreditation has been optional and has varied from setting to setting. The standards have changed from year to year and have never fully addressed the issue of professional competence.

Finally, we must consider the role of the nurse working in the treatment center. Some treatment centers will hire any licensed nurse, regardless of his or her ability and background. Sometimes these nurses need or have just finished chemical dependency treatment themselves. This is a problem for the nurse in treatment because of the possibility that the treatment may be compromised. And treatment by an addicted nurse provides a poor role model. The encounter with a colleague working in the treatment program should be therapeutic. Nurses as caregivers in treatment centers could assume a primary role in all therapeutic activities of the program. They should have the education and experience to fill such a role. See Chapter 11 for more discussion on education for nurses working in treatment.

CHAPTER 5

USING DRUGS FOR MONITORING AND RECOVERY

ANTABUSE® AND TREXAN®

Disulfiram (Antabuse®) and naltrexone (Trexan®) may be suggested or even required as part of a treatment or monitoring program. Neither drug should be used as the sole form of treatment. If well understood and used thoughtfully, each can effectively supplement other approaches. Each drug has a specific application: Antabuse is for alcohol and Trexan for opiates. Neither drug will affect the addiction symptoms of cocaine or other stimulants, marijuana, sedatives and tranquilizers. If the nurse has been abusing more than one class of drugs simultaneously, the usefulness of Antabuse and Trexan will be limited.

Antabuse

Antabuse has been available since its accidental discovery during World War II. It is taken orally, usually in a dose of 250 to 500 mg once a day. Antabuse suspends but does not dissolve in water, so if it is given under supervision during a monitoring program it is usually pulverized and mixed with fruit juice.[1]

The effects of Antabuse are straightforward. If adequate amounts of alcohol and Antabuse are simultaneously present in the body, sickness results. The reaction usually includes flushing, tachycardia, nausea, vomiting, headache, a drop in blood pressure, and complaints of "just feeling awful." People who have experienced an Antabuse reaction usually are very reluctant to repeat it. Many people experiment by sipping alcohol to see if the Antabuse really does work; they are usually quickly convinced. The side effects of Antabuse may include allergic reactions or an annoying, unpleasant garlic breath odor. Death has been reported in the past in connection with the alcohol–Antabuse reaction but this is rare, and usually associated with higher maintenance doses than are common today.

The potential for an Antabuse reaction with alcohol will continue for two to three days. Once Antabuse has been absorbed, a person will not be able to drink for that period without experiencing illness. Antabuse works. Failure may be attributed only to insufficient dosage or total lack of injection. Antabuse can buy time and it will guarantee sobriety while it is in effect. It can help the user and the caregiver relax and feel more secure with each other, thus obviating the need for spying and surreptitious breath sniffing. Antabuse will have little effect on other addictive drugs, although a minimal slowing of their rate of metabolism has been noted with some addictive drugs. An excellent discussion of the pros and cons, methods, and complications of Antabuse use can be found in *Alcoholism, A Practical Treatment Guide* (Gitlow & Peyser, 1980). We strongly recommend this text to anyone using or administering Antabuse.

---

[1]Tablets may be concealed in a patient's cheek pouch and later discarded. Other tablets can be substituted for the Antabuse if the addicted nurse monitors the supply. Sometimes another tablet is hidden in the mouth and substituted for the Antabuse. Rarely, a person may swallow a little oil to delay gastric emptying, take the Antabuse, then promptly induce vomiting. If the alcoholic nurse is using Antabuse voluntarily and is not being monitored by someone else, these subterfuges need not be considered.

Trexan

Trexan is used to prevent enjoyment of opiates. Whereas Antabuse combined with alcohol causes the drinker to feel miserable, Trexan combined with opiates causes no illness. It does, however, eliminate the pleasurable effects of opiates by acting as a blocker. When a narcotic is injected, nothing much happens. Trexan can be taken orally and is usually given under supervision three times per week. Dosage is 50 mg a day, so a person can take 100 mg (two tablets) every other day or 150 mg (three tablets) every third day. Trexan therapy should not be instituted while a patient is still using opiates as it will produce immediate withdrawal.

METHADONE

The methadone maintenance technique of addiction treatment has a long and controversial history. Few health care professionals have successfully sustained methadone maintenance. We stress that methadone maintenance should be considered only for those whose chemical dependency is limited to opiates since it cannot be expected to counteract other drugs.

Neither Antabuse nor Trexan is regarded as a drug of addiction. Methadone, however, is a narcotic, is diverted, and has illicit street users. It can create physical dependency leading to a significant withdrawal syndrome if it is abruptly discontinued. An overdose can kill.

Methadone is substituted for opiates like Demerol® morphine, and heroin, whose action is rapid and whose effect is of relatively short duration. It can be given once a day orally. Its effect is sustained, therefore the user is spared the peaks and valley of sudden highs and rapid withdrawals with accompanying discomfort and drug hunger. At regular "maintenance" dosage, its presence overwhelms the effects of additional opiates the nurse may take.

Methadone is also used for brief periods during acute withdrawal from other opiates. It has also been used to stabilize a patient before weaning to drug-free status. The weaning process is difficult for most narcotic addicts and we have little information about the success of this approach for health care professionals. A few nurses have sustained methadone maintenance regimens for indefinite periods, with no specific tapering-off goal. This continues to be a controversial approach.

We repeat that methadone is for opiate addiction only. This point has also been stressed by Vincent Dole and Marie Nyswander, the physicians who pioneered the use of methadone. And we do not agree with those who believe that prolonged use of opiates permanently alters the brain such that permanent abstinence is impossible. Even after prolonged use of massive amounts of pure narcotic drugs, many physicians and nurses have achieved total, sustained freedom from those drugs. Pessimism about full recovery is unnecessary and unproductive. Most treatment programs today set goals of total abstinence and few employers or liability carriers will want a nurse returning to work while still on a narcotic.

Psychotropic Drugs

It is inappropriate to assume that one is mentally ill because one has become addicted; likewise it is wrong to assume that chemical dependency protects one from mental illnesses. Alcoholics and other addicts may have phobias, panic attacks, and affective disorders or may be schizophrenic. We have stressed that diagnoses should be made after the confounding effects of alcohol and other drug use and the turbulent effects of prolonged withdrawal have passed. At this point a small number of people will be diagnosed with independent psychiatric problems for which psychotropic drugs might be prescribed. But how will the use of psychotropic drugs affect the individual and his or her relationship with the members of AA or other mutual support groups?

AA has had a long and rather stormy relationship with health care professionals. Its members have earnestly tried not to practice medicine and to defer to physicians, only to find too many drugs dispensed by caregivers with little or no knowledge of chemical dependency. This situation has resulted in relapse, the development of additional addictions, and often, tragedy and death. Understandably many addicted nurses become wary, suspicious, and mistrustful. They often have more knowledge than the health care establishment that rejected them or treated them ineptly while dismissing AA as little more than folk medicine.

Although AA is careful to recognize its unique role as well as its strengths and limitations, individual groups and members have their own attitudes and rigidities. Some will immediately reject psychiatric help. Others will resist mood-altering drugs. Many are cautiously neutral.

Unfortunately, AA members may not be able to differentiate between hazardous and helpful drugs. Some members have urged other members to stop taking Antabuse in the belief that it was a tranquilizer. One member persuaded her protegé to stop taking thyroid medication because she herself had once inappropriately combined an amphetamine with a thyroid capsule from a "diet doctor." Others have rejected the use of lithium and phenothiazines, even when these drugs were necessary and appropriately administered.

If psychotropic drugs are truly necessary, the patient must be taught to understand their action and side-effects, and to anticipate the level of support from AA or other similar support groups. We must be sensitive to AA's attitude and explain the need for the drug and its prescribed length of treatment. A distinction must be made between using the drug to treat the chemical dependency and using it to treat a parallel but separate problem. Treatment with a psychotropic drug may complicate the nurse's relationship with the support group, but the apparent contradiction may be understood and resolved with sophistication.

SEDATIVES AND TRANQUILIZERS

The treatment issues for tranquilizers are more complex. Because addicts may be prone to addiction to other drugs, administration of mood-changing drugs with potential for dependency should be avoided if possible. Except for their appropriate but brief use in early withdrawal, sedatives and tranquilizers (including alcohol) should virtually never be used. They do encourage sleep and alleviate anxiety, but both have pitfalls. Soporifics are effective for only a few days unless the dose is increased, and sleep is even more difficult to attain after they are discontinued. Even in recommended dosage, benzodiazapine tranquilizer use has resulted in significant withdrawal problems. The combination of alcohol and benzodiazapines is the leading cause of fatal poisonings in hospital emergency rooms in the United States. In many cases, the tranquilizers had been innocently prescribed for unsuspected alcoholics whose problem should have been diagnosed.

AMPHETAMINES AND ANTIDEPRESSANTS

Amphetamines are no longer readily prescribed, so addicts often obtain them illegally. Antidepressants, particularly Elavil®, are more problematic. Addicts who have discovered the tranquilizing, sleep-inducing side effect of Elavil have used it to their detriment. Antidepressants are sometimes indicated, but they should be prescribed with caution for short time periods only.

ANTIPSYCHOTICS

Lithium and the phenothiazines are less likely to be casually prescribed. With the omnipresent risk of lawsuits there is little enthusiasm for risking toxicity, tardive dyskinesia, or impotence unless there is a real indication for prescription. Levels of lithium and electrolytes must be monitored since the toxic and therapeutic range is close. Early enthusiasm for lithium prescription for alcoholics has waned.

WORDS OF CAUTION

In addition to the potential physical consequences, the risk of dependency, or the complication of support group affiliation, prescription of drugs can have a psychologic effect on recovery. Chemically dependent people may believe that there is a chemical solution for human problems. When we prescribe psychotropics, we reinforce that idea. With drug therapy, there is much less apparent need to change habits, attitudes, friends, or lifestyle. Why spend time at AA meetings discussing the hard work of growing up and facing the world without chemical consolation if a prescription drug will solve the problem? If drugs are prescribed, there is a subtle message that one cannot be expected or trusted to exist without them. At the same time, palliative use of drugs can undermine the need to make the major behavioral commitments necessary to change. It is for these reasons that some of us feel that even M&Ms could be dangerous to alcoholics and other addicts if they were sorted by color and dispensed by a pharmacist.

Drug therapy can be effective in managing chemical dependency. Drugs are useful during withdrawal, for pain, for concomitant mental illness, and to interfere with the reinforcing effects of alcohol or opiates. They should be used with respect and a clear understanding of chemical dependency, the psychiatric considerations independent of the addiction, the individual nurse, and the social, political, and occupational setting.

CHAPTER 6

REENTRY

Reentry into the workplace is the ultimate goal of successful intervention and treatment of chemical dependency. In fact, vocational rehabilitation is a vital component of recovery. A successful reentry benefits the recovering nurse and the employer as well. The recovering nurse retains job, income, and self-respect, and the employer retains an experienced employee. The employer will want assurance that patients will receive competent care from a nurse whose performance is unimpaired by drug use. The employer's reluctance to reemploy a recovering nurse is grounded in the fear of relapse into chemical dependency and consequent danger to patients.

HIRING A RECOVERING NURSE

Given a choice of applicants, most nursing administrators would prefer not to hire a nurse whom they know has been actively alcoholic or dependent on other drugs. However, several factors should prevent such discrimination. Federal law specifies that alcohol and drug dependent people are included in the category of handicapped individuals and are thus protected from discriminatory employment practices.

This means that the employer must base employment and promotion decisions solely on the potential for job performance. A prior history of chemical dependency alone, if there is a current sustained record of recovery, is not sufficient reason for discrimination. Furthermore, interview questions and tests must be used consistently for all applicants, and these selection techniques may not be used to identify a disability (in this case, chemical dependency). Only a disability that would interfere with job performance may be identified and used as grounds for rejection.

Confidentiality of Records

Federal law protects the chemical dependent by assuring confidentiality of any records of treatment received for alcohol or other drug dependency. No employer can access a chemical dependent's record of treatment without that person's written permission. In addition, many states have laws to strengthen the existing federal statutes. Recovering nurses are protected from discrimination due to their disability just as recovering chemical dependents in the general population are protected.

Despite confidentiality of treatment records, nurses are subject to the requirements of licensing agencies, which may reveal a chemical dependency history. If, for instance, the licensing agency has placed sanctions on a nurse's license, this action becomes a matter of public record. Furthermore, many states require applicants for a new or reciprocal license to answer questions about their past experience with alcohol or other drug dependency and/or treatment. An employer can obtain from state board records information on past disciplinary action as well as nurses' responses to chemical dependency queries. While the employer cannot legally use this information to discriminate against a potential employee without evidence of continued dependency, anecdotal accounts from recovering nurses indicate that many have experienced discrimination in hiring following investigations by potential employers as well as voluntary personal admissions.

Hiring Discrimination

During a job interview, one nurse told the interviewer that she had "a handicap." She was told, "We'll talk about that later, we need you in the ICU." While filling out employment forms, she told the personnel staff person that she had a handicap and again was told that it would be handled "later." Finally, during the pre-employment physical, she explained that she had been chemically dependent but was now in recovery. She was called to the nursing administrator's office and told, "We can't have people like you working here." In another case, a nurse worked to everyone's satisfaction until the eighty-eighth day of a 90-day probationary period. She then shared her recovery experience with another nurse on her unit. The next day she was fired.

Many nurses are forced into lying to conceal the past. Some nurses report that they lie or evade questions regarding past chemical dependency treatment on job applications because they know it is an illegal topic and because they fear being rejected regardless of their capabilities. The "catch 22" is that if they refuse to answer the question, the employer may become suspicious and not hire them anyway (ostensibly for other reasons).

Successful Reentry

Despite understandable hesitance by the employers to hire recovering chemical dependents, studies of recovery rates from chemical dependency indicate that successful reentry to nursing practice can indeed be achieved, especially with effective intervention, treatment, and support (Bissell & Haberman, 1984; Hutchinson, 1986; Sullivan, 1987a). One study that focused on physicians found that their rate of abstinence after treatment was higher than that of other people (Morse, Martin, Swenson, & Niven, 1984). This higher recovery rate was, in part, attributed to the threat of license revocation. Although sufficient data on specific recovery rates for nurses is not available, it could be assumed that nurses' motivation for recovery would be similar to that of physicians, assuming the same provision for aftercare and monitoring.

In the best-case scenario, the recovering nurse would return rapidly to the former job after completing primary treatment. In reality, this scenario may not be possible. For instance, the former job may require rotating shift assignments that would interfere with regular attendance at continuing care sessions or support group meetings. If the job duties require the nurse to administer the drug of choice and other mood-altering drugs of addiction, the easy access to the drugs may be unwise at this early stage. The key to resolution of these potential threats to recovery is careful and individualized reentry planning, along with ongoing monitoring to ensure prompt detection of a relapse.

Planning for Reentry

When the nurse is recovering from drug addiction, several factors should be considered in the reentry plan. If the nurse will be unsupervised for many working hours or has unrestricted access to the addictive drug, most experts in rehabilitation suggest that a period of time elapse before returning the nurse to that particular situation. Although forfeiting one's chosen job and/or one's preferred clinical area seems a harsh penalty for a returning nurse, it must be reiterated that the nurse is recovering from a life-threatening chronic disease. Sustained recovery means lifelong vigilance; we cannot afford to underestimate the power of the disease. A change in specialty may be a small price to pay for one's health and future.

Most employers reassign returning drug dependent nurses to areas with little or no access to addictive drugs. The change in assignment may be permanent if the nurse agrees to change career direction, or it may be temporary for a period of six months to two years. While most nursing positions do involve administration of mood-altering medication, units like the nursery, physical rehabilitation, and the education department provide minimal access to these drugs. Supervisory jobs do not necessarily require administration of narcotics. If the nurse formerly held an administrative position, such as head nurse, he or she may be allowed to return to that position.

When alternative assignments are not available, or if the nurse lacks the necessary experience or credentials to fill another position, there may be a return to the former unit but with special provisions. For example, other staff in the unit would be asked to temporarily administer mood-altering medications to the recovering nurse's patients. This allows the nurse to return to patient care without access to narcotics. In these cases, the cooperating staff members are generally told that the recovering nurse has a disability and cannot administer narcotics. This disability is no different from a physical problem. This arrangement generally involves little additional time and effort from the rest of the staff. Obviously there is no way to conceal the reason for such a limitation, and this necessary evil must be accepted by the recovering nurse. (See also Chapter 10 regarding ethical issues.) When the recovering nurse, the supervisor, the treatment counselor, and employee assistance program staff believe that direct access to drugs is no longer a threat to recovery, the nurse may be allowed to administer controlled substances.

Monitoring for Continued Abstinence

Monitoring the nurse's recovery is critical for the employer *and* for the recovering nurse. During monitoring, the employer is assured that the nurse is not practicing while drug impaired, thus protecting patients from incompetent care and the institution from potential liability. Furthermore, the monitoring process provides the recovering nurse with documentation of sustained recovery, so that there is little danger of false accusations and threats to continued employment. A nurse with a known history of addiction will be the most likely suspect when drugs are missing. Proof of guilt is easier to produce than proof of innocence. Without documentation, the latter is nearly impossible.

This monitoring process is important regardless of the source of the addiction. The person may be dependent on a narcotic that was diverted from the workplace or obtained elsewhere (alcohol, prescription drugs, or "street drugs"). The goal is to document continued abstinence and continued progress in therapy.

Monitoring Methods

To reenter the workplace, it is customary that the recovering nurse sign a document specifying expected behaviors. An important aspect of monitoring includes documentation of these behaviors as outlined in a return-to-work contract (Figure 6–1). Expected behaviors may include the following:

O Consistant attendance at specific mutual help groups such as AA or NA or a nurses' support group (if available)

O Documentation of continued treatment as recommended by a therapist

_____ Hospital Employee Assistance Program
Agreement Between Employee and _____ Hospital

I, _____ , agree to the following conditions upon my continuing employment at _____ Hospital. These conditions will apply for a period of two years, beginning on _____ and ending on _____ .

1. If it should be determined that I am using any mood-altering chemicals (except with the agreement of my therapist and under the direction of a physician who will keep the Employee Assistance Program informed as to reason and specific period of time), I will be immediately terminated and reported to the State Board of Nursing.

2. I agree to cooperate in any random urine check requested by_____ Hospital. The results will be sent to the Employee Assistance Program. If at any time mood-altering substances are found, my employment will be terminated immediately and I will be reported to the State Board of Nursing.

3. I agree to follow the prescribed program of aftercare, including attendance in AA. I will be responsible for providing documentation of attendance to the Employee Assistance Program and if I do not comply, either in attendance and/ or documentation, my employment will be terminated immediately and I will be reported to the State Board of Nursing.

4. If I should voluntarily terminate from _____ Hospital, I agree to keep the Employee Assistance Program informed as to my compliance with prescribed program of aftercare, my address and place of employment. I further agree to inform my new employer of my condition and request my new employer to keep the Employee Assistance Program at _____ Hospital informed of my progress. Unless other arrangements are made which are mutually agreeable to the new employer and the Employee Assistance Program at_____ Hospital, and if the above conditions are not met I will be reported to the State Board of Nursing.

These four conditions have been read and agreed upon by:

_____   _____
(Employee signature)   (Date)
In the presence of:

_____   _____
(Director of Nursing—_____ Hospital)   (Date)

_____   _____
(EAP Coordinator—_____ Hospital)   (Date)

Figure 6-1. Return-to-work contract. (Courtesy of The Jewish Hospital of St. Louis.)

O Regular sessions with an employee assistance counselor. If the institution does not have an employee assistance program, a knowledgeable and concerned administrator can be designated as the contact person.

O Actions required of the nurse and the employer if the nurse voluntarily resigns from the institution (eg, nurse reports regularly to former employer and informs new employer of his/her status). The contract also states the consequences if the terms of the contract and its proposed duration are not honored. The health care institution has the right to terminate the nurse's employment and to report the nurse to the state board of nursing.

The nurse provides documentation of attendance at AA or NA meetings by obtaining a signed statement of attendance. Reports on the nurse's progress are provided to the administrator or supervisor on a regular basis by the employee assistance counselor and/or treatment facility staff. The report need not include intimate personal details but should indicate cooperation with treatment in general. When possible the treatment and monitoring roles should be separated. Occasionally Antabuse® or Trexan® may be administered under careful supervision. More common are random urine screens or blood tests, for reassurance of both the employer and the nurse. Since the employer schedules the test without prior notice to the nurse, the supervisor is assured that a relapsing nurse cannot prepare for the test by temporarily abstaining from alcohol or drugs. Random drug screens, conducted frequently over a long time period, also help the recovering nurse in proving abstinence. They must be truly random and the collection of the specimen carefully performed.

Drug/alcohol monitoring should be handled privately and confidentially. To collect the specimen, the appropriate supervisor should ask the nurse to provide an immediate urine sample. A staff member should actually observe the voiding of the specimen. The sample is then sent to a laboratory previously designated for this purpose. Often this is done in the employer's hospital, however, arrangements can be made with an outside laboratory. The urine specimen should be tested for the presence of alcohol or any other mood-altering drugs and the results sent to a specified person. To assure confidentiality, some administrators use a "John Doe" order or a code number for identification and arrange for the results to be sent directly to the nursing administrator or employee assistance counselor. To avoid opportunity for tampering, a "chain of custody" should be established to collect, label, and transport the specimen to the post office or the laboratory.

The laboratory analysis may be paid for by the nurse, borne by the institution, or the nurse and institution may share the expense. Because of the expense and the complexity of arranging drug screening tests, many administrators forego this method of monitoring. It is, however, the most reliable method of assuring ongoing abstinence and should be used for monitoring whenever possible.

Drug testing should not be the sole factor or carry more weight in determining recovery than other elements of the agreement. For example, if a nurse's job performance is deteriorating but urine tests remain negative for drugs, the nurse might still be terminated. In another case, a reliable positive urine in the presence of adequate job performance may be cause for job termination *or* an immediate admission for residential treatment. Drug testing will be discussed further in Chapter 9.

Contingency Contracting

Contingency contracting was first described by Thomas Crowley, MD, of Colorado. The "contingency" is a real or strongly suspected return to drug or alcohol use. The nurse signs a letter to the appropriate disciplinary board which says in effect, "If you receive this letter, it will mean that I have returned to my drug(s) of dependency and I am therefore requesting that my license be immediately revoked or suspended." The letter is undated and remains in the custody of the monitor. If there is relapse, the monitor dates and delivers the letter to the board. This encourages rapid action in case of trouble. Whereas other procedures may take months, the potential use of this procedure reassures reluctant employers that if necessary they can proceed without long delays and complicated legal battles. It is a strong measure and the monitor must use this procedure only in accordance with the agreement under which it was drawn.

Who Is Responsible for Monitoring Activities?

Monitoring is the responsibility of management and should not involve other staff unless their assistance is required. If staff members know about the nurse's addiction, they will have concerns about how to "handle" the returning nurse. They will wonder if they should watch for signs of alcohol or other drug use or observe the nurse when he or she is near the narcotics cabinet. It may be helpful to hold a meeting to educate the staff. In any case, staff should be assured that management is responsible for monitoring and supervision that the returning nurse should be treated as normally as possible. The best explanation is straightforward: The nurse is recovering from a chronic, but treatable, disease.

The nursing administrator may delegate monitoring responsibility to a subordinate administrator or to the nurse's immediate supervisor. It is essential that one person coordinate all monitoring activities. Expectations of the monitor should be delineated and agreement reached as to exactly how to handle a real or suspected relapse. All documentation from reporting personnel should be kept in a confidential file, along with test reports for alcohol and other drug use.

What If There Is a Relapse?

The monitor must understand what to do if evidence of alcohol or other drug use is discovered. A relapsing nurse *must* be removed from patient care activities immediately and nursing administration informed. A conference should be held with all involved parties—counselors, supervisors, the administrator, and the nurse. Often a brief relapse signals the need for additional support or counseling and does not indicate a permanent return to drug dependency. The nurse's therapist should be consulted immediately. The nurse might be advised to return to residential treatment, to meet more frequently with a counselor, or to attend AA or NA meetings more often. An alternative monitoring regimen might be instituted. The nurse may be removed from patient care for a period of time or given a medical leave of absence. If the employer, after thoughtful consultation with the treatment and counseling staff, believes that the nurse is unlikely to remain abstinent, employment should be terminated and the nurse reported to the state board of nursing. Issues of disciplinary action are discussed in Chapter 8.

Should Nurses' Support Groups Participate in Monitoring?

The role of nurses' chemical dependency support groups during recovery monitoring is controversial. A support group's leader and its members follow the progress of the recovering nurse and may know if the nurse is using drugs again. They have a responsibility to protect patients if the nurse is practicing while impaired. The purpose of the group, however, is to offer support and assistance with recovery. If the nurse "slips" (uses alcohol or other drugs), it is the group's responsibility to help a member regain sobriety. It would be difficult, if not impossible, for the nurse to confide in the group when he or she knows that the group will report the event to an employer or state board of nursing.

This dilemma may be resolved by separating the monitoring and support activities. For example, the Georgia Nurses' Association has an established assistance program for nurses. A volunteer may serve as nurse advocate *or* monitor. The advocate acts as liaison between the nurse and the employer or the state board of nursing and provides the nurse with referrals to treatment and other services. The monitor documents the nurse's employment and recovery status for all involved parties (employer, state board). Both roles are perceived by the Georgia Nurses' Association as necessary for a comprehensive assistance program.

When expectations are understood at the beginning of the process, these different functional roles can operate effectively, albeit not without periodic ethical dilemmas. A monitor is not a best friend. A therapist is not an enforcer. Nurses' support groups usually refuse to participate in monitoring unless the members believe that patient safety is endangered. They may recommend that all monitoring be the responsibility of the employer and/or the state board of nursing. An active nurses' support group in Minneapolis has maintained the AA practice of nondisclosure of membership since its inception in 1981. Other groups have had serious disputes and some have disbanded when the group "betrayed" a member by reporting a relapse. If relapses may be reported by support groups, only the successful are likely to be candid about their progress. However, some relapses pose a distinct threat to patient safety. This ethical and legal dilemma remains, and patient safety, the nurse's recovery, and the long-term reputation of the group must be evaluated on a case-by-case basis. For more information about nurses' support groups, see Chapter 4.

Respect for Privacy

If a nurse has been absent from work while in inpatient treatment, other staff will wonder why. Often, however, staff members are aware of the nurse's condition because of past behavior. Nurses' explanations of their restricted access to drugs vary a great deal. Some nurses do not want to discuss the situation with their colleagues, so only those that need to know are aware of the restrictions. We may assume that the reasons for such secrecy are the guilt and shame so many nurses experience. There are other considerations, however, that are frequently feared by the nurse, such as blame for others' mistakes or exclusion from social activities.

Some nurses feel comfortable discussing their illness and recovery with anyone when it seems appropriate. A nurse in recovery for about six months, whose access to narcotics was still restricted, said, "I'm a drug addict. I denied it for years. It's simply too complicated for me to find excuses for anything any longer. I'll get the keys (narcotics) back someday, but for now I'm still a damned good nurse and if anyone wants to talk about me or any part of this experience, it's okay with me. Maybe it will help someone else."

It is inappropriate for a manager to inform the staff of a nurse's treatment, however, some explanation must be given. It is best to discuss the situation with the nurse and treatment counselor. Some recovering nurses report a leave of absence for medical or personal reasons and others share their recovery experience with their colleagues. Although the degree of disclosure should remain the nurse's decision, full confidentiality may be impossible when the staff's assistance is necessary to restrict drug access. The nurse's dignity is important. Control and autonomy during the decision-making process help keep it intact.

CHAPTER 7

SOURCES OF HELP FOR THE CHEMICALLY DEPENDENT NURSE

ASSISTANCE NEEDS

A nurse who has been coping with a chemical dependency problem is likely to need a variety of additional assistance and support services. For nurses who have been involved in diversion of drugs other than alcohol, there are legal, career, and ethical dilemmas to face. Depending on the circumstances, the situation may be reported to the state board of nursing or criminal charges may be instituted. Employers and state boards of nursing must make public safety their first priority and ensure that no nurse cares for patients while he or she is in an impaired condition. After recovery, the nurse must be able to demonstrate not only freedom from the effects of drugs, but the likelihood of remaining drug-free.

Legal Assistance

Drug theft is a felony, so criminal charges may also be pending. In this case the nurse will need skilled legal advice. Board of nursing procedures and criminal court are very different. While it may benefit a recovering nurse to reveal the full story of addiction to the board, the same testimony in criminal court may provoke legal consequences that endanger licensure. Many recovering nurses seek assistance in evaluating the complicated implications of disciplinary activities.

One recovering nurse left her state of origin for treatment and remained in the new location to earn a master's degree. She decided to stay out of clinical practice for a while and let other nurses get to know her while she demonstrated her ability to function well as a student and to remain drug-free. That done and recommendations in hand, she sought a license through reciprocity. Her original license had not been in jeopardy and was still valid. Her new state refused her a license; its policy for addicts in recovery who wished to transfer from other states required a demonstrated ability to work as nurses, not students, for at least a year. There was legal assistance available to members of the state nurses' association but the assistance was limited to association members and one could not become a member unless eligible for a license. Finally an attorney (who was an alcoholic in recovery) was able to resolve this particular case but was not able to set precedent for others.

Financial Assistance

Another critical problem is the financial burden of the treatment process. Many nurses exclude health insurance coverage for addictive illnesses from their basic policies, in the belief that addiction could not affect them or their families. Mistaken beliefs about the disease lead both insurers and policy holders to resist coverage in an attempt to keep the cost of premiums down. Research indicates, however, that treatment of alcoholism results in cost savings (Berry, 1981). When alcoholics are treated for the dependency itself, rather than for its secondary health consequences, insurers actually save money. Furthermore, health expenditures decrease for the nuclear family as well as for the alcoholic (Holder, Blose, & Gasiorowski, 1985). Additional research is necessary to determine whether or not these cost savings apply to drug addictions other than alcoholism.

When a nurse's employer-provided insurance policy does cover chemical dependency treatment, there may be loss of coverage if intervention is not handled properly. If the employer fires the nurse abruptly, the necessary medical coverage may be lost at the time when it is most needed. Even though federal legislation now requires that employees, and in some cases, their families, be allowed to continue coverage after leaving employment, the cost of that coverage may not be affordable without a job. One solution to this problem is to keep the nurse employed and on medical leave until primary treatment is completed. Thus the nurse can have access to the necessary treatment and the employer protects patient safety by removing the nurse from the workplace. Unfortunately, the nurse is usually incapable of negotiating or even suggesting this compromise. The firing itself is traumatic, and may leave the nurse unprepared to consider or plan for treatment.

In coping with these and other problems, the chemically dependent nurse may need the assistance of a professional who is sensitive to the impending difficulties and knowledgeable about the variety of available solutions.

SOURCES OF ASSISTANCE

Assistance programs for chemically dependent nurses are designed to intervene when professional functioning is impaired, to provide treatment referral services, to provide support and encouragement during the difficult early recovery period, and to monitor reentry to the workplace. The primary role of most structured assistance programs is to assist with intervention and reentry, however, ongoing support may be offered. More often, the nurse is referred to a nurses' support group if possible. The conflict between the goals of support services and monitoring functions are discussed in Chapters 4 and 6. Some programs provide extensive support services, while others limit their focus to education of the health care community. Activities vary depending on the resources available, the stage of program development, and attitude toward the appropriate degree of monitoring to be included in recovery.

State Boards of Nursing

The primary role of the state board is to administer licensure and disciplinary actions, but some state boards are also providing assistance to chemically dependent nurses. State board assistance programs are authorized by legislative action. Known as diversion legislation, these laws "divert" nurses out of the disciplinary process if they agree to obtain treatment and enter a program that monitors their recovery. (The term diversion has no relation to "drug diversion," which refers to stealing drugs from the workplace.) Under the diversion laws, if the nurse at any time fails to adhere to the agreed-upon plan, the case reverts to the regular disciplinary procedure. Diversion legislation varies from state to state. To date, Florida, California, Texas, and New Mexico have passed diversion legislation. In Texas, the renewal licensure fee for nurses was increased to cover the cost; in California funding is provided from licensing fees but there have been no recent increases in the fees; in Florida and New Mexico, funds are allocated by state appropriations.

The Florida State Board of Nursing has established an "impaired nurse program" (Penny, 1986). To ensure eligibility for this program a nurse must: (a) request a leave of absence from employment to enter treatment, (b) want to enter treatment, hold an active license, but not be employed in nursing; (c) have been confronted with evidence of chemical substance and agree to treatment; (d) currently be in a treatment program; or (e) be impaired due to a physical or mental condition and participating in a rehabilitation program. Referrals may also be made by an employer. After substantiation of a genuine problem, an intervention conference is planned. The administrator and a local resource person designated by the state board of nursing (treatment staff, employee assistance counselor) confront the nurse, who is given the choice of admission to treatment or job termination. If the nurse successfully completes treatment, follows a prescribed regimen of recovery (AA attendance, random urine or blood screens, regular reports to the board), and has no other disciplinary action against the nursing license, there will be no further action as long as recovery progress is maintained for a two-year period. Unsatisfactory progress or noncompliance will result in dismissal from the program and initiation of disciplinary proceedings by the state's Department of Professional Regulation.

The state board may be empowered to administer the program. It may hire its own staff experts or contract with an outside organization or person to run it. It may also refer the nurse to a state nurses' association program (see next section) or an employee assistance program. A model for diversion legislation has been developed by the National Nurses Society on Addictions (See Appendix F).

State Nurses' Association Peer Assistance Programs

Some states established assistance programs for chemically dependent nurses prior to 1982, but the adoption that year of a national resolution by the American Nurses' Association (ANA) House of Delegates to assist impaired nurses and the subsequent monograph on development of assistance programs (American Nurses' Association, 1984) encouraged more state associations to initiate program planning. This resolution may be found in Appendix B.

The majority of nurses' associations have either established programs of assistance or are in the process of discussing such programs. These programs are usually developed by a committee of members designated by the board of directors of the state association to develop plans for an assistance program. The committees are often composed of nurses who are concerned about their colleagues and nurses who are in recovery themselves. Because members are colleagues, programs are called peer assistance programs.

A typical peer assistance program involves a series of contacts with people designated to provide assistance. (See Figure 7-1 for model of typical program.) Contact begins with a publicized telephone number and a procedure for referring callers for assistance. This number could be the state nurses' association office or a separate number specifically dedicated to the program. Calls may be taken by a secretary who requests a number where the call can be returned. The secretary then notifies a specified contact to return the call. The contacts are usually determined by geographical proximity to the caller. The contact person answers questions and makes an appointment to meet to plan an intervention.

Calls may be received from the chemically dependent nurse or from a concerned co-worker, friend, or family member. Or an employer may call and ask for assistance with an intervention. Most programs require a second party to substantiate the concerns unless the nurse is self-referring or the employer makes the request for assistance. The gathering of documentation can be implemented by securing the names of other people who are aware of the nurse's drugs/alcohol use and asking them to substantiate the reported behaviors. If the caller insists on remaining anonymous to the addicted nurse, the need for verification of the report is essential.

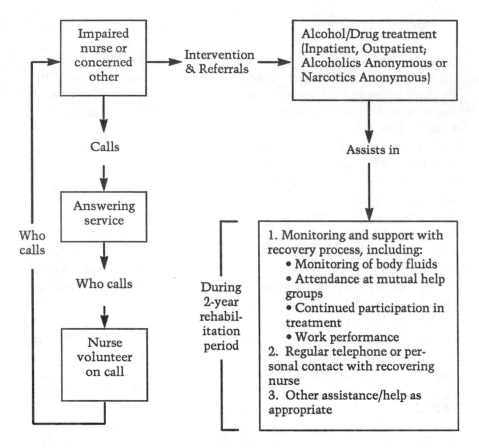

Figure 7-1. Model for peer assistance program.

Volunteers are selected from various areas of the state, with careful attention to the qualifications necessary to serve as intervenors and counselors to chemically dependent nurses. Some of these qualifications include:

o A background in psychiatric or mental health (education or experience) with particular emphasis on addictive illnesses

o Previous work (employment or volunteer) with alcoholic or drug-dependent clients

o Participation in a co-dependency program such as Al-Anon

o Personal experience as a nurse in recovery with a one- to two-year
   period of abstinence and active AA/NA participation

Volunteers are trained in intervention and assistance techniques.
They are also taught about addiction in nursing, the special problems
nurses encounter, and referral options to appropriate treatment and
mutual-help groups. Experiential learning is especially useful in helping participants role-play typical crisis situations. The sensitivity and
vulnerability of the nurse who is using drugs or is in the beginning
stages of withdrawal must be given special consideration. Peer assistance programs should include regular meetings to help the volunteers
cope with emerging problems as well as with the stress of assisting colleagues in trouble.

Employee Assistance Programs

Many hospitals and other health care institutions now have in-house
programs for chemical dependency. The programs may be part of an
EAP or under contract with an EAP provider. In some areas, in-house
and contract services are combined. The Association of Labor-Management Administrators and Consultants in Alcoholism (ALMACA) is an
organization of alcoholism experts who work in a variety of health care
settings. Despite their name, their services address other drug problems and personal difficulties that may affect an employee's job.

EAPs in hospitals are usually based on well-accepted industry
models that are operational in most Fortune 500 companies. Many
EAPs, both in health care settings and in industry, are run by nurses.

Hospital EAPs generally set policy for all employees—professional
and nonprofessional, upper management, and support staff. EAPs
provide or arrange for education, outreach, case finding, referral to
treatment, and monitoring services. EAPs focus on employees' work
performances rather than their private lives, unless and until they
intrude on the job.

The advantage of an EAP is that the hospital can provide staff
salaries for its operation, rather than relying on volunteers as do many
peer support programs. The disadvantage is that since the EAP focuses
only on impaired job performance, early cases are neglected until
observable interference with work occurs. Observable impact on the

job often occurs late in the development of the disease. Some EAPs notify families that their service is available and invite them to use it, thus allowing the possibility of an earlier intervention.

Another problem with employer-run programs is that those in positions of influence can "deal themselves out"; ie, administrators who have a chemical dependency problem can continue their denial and skirt the assistance/intervention process. If too many department heads or other top administrators decide that the EAP is only for middle- and lower-level personnel, the program's strength and accomplishments will be limited.

Another problem in developing EAPs in health care is the lack of recognition of the significant value and impact of this kind of program. Most practicing physicians (including psychiatrists) are unaware of the expertise of EAP counselors and the extremely effective pressure that the workplace can apply to encourage an employee to seek help. (Kornblum, 1987). Basic information on EAPs is available in a number of books and pamphlets from the National Institute on Alcohol Abuse and Alcoholism (NIAAA), local National Council on Alcohol (NCA) affiliates, ALMACA, and specialty publishers in the chemical dependency field. These addresses are listed in Appendix E. For more information about employee assistance programs, refer to *Alcoholism and Drug Abuse in the Workplace: Employee Assistance Programs* (Scanlon, 1986). Appendix G presents a model EAP program for hospitals.

Other Sources of Assistance

Private organizations and entrepreneurs also offer assistance to chemically dependent nurses. In Tampa, Florida, for instance, the Tampa Area Hospital Council for some years provided intervention and referral services for chemically dependent nurses. They also provided education about chemical dependency to local hospitals, nurses, and administrators. Unlike the state nurses' associations' peer assistance programs, yet similar to board of nursing programs, paid staff, rather than volunteers, provided services. The member hospitals in the Tampa Area Hospital Council each contributed the necessary funds.

In addition to hospital-sponsored programs, services are provided by an increasing number of private entrepreneurs. Many of these businesses are started by nurses. Some are well prepared for the work. Others are self-styled experts who may have personal recovery experience and a general mental health background, but lack expertise in the field of chemical dependency intervention and treatment. It is important to investigate carefully the preparation and credentials of would-be assistance providers (see Chapter 4).

FUNDING OF ASSISTANCE PROGRAMS

Industry recognized long ago that running a good EAP paid off handsomely, but it also had to admit that it required an investment. To care for several thousand employees in a large plant, identify the ones who were ill, and provide treatment and recovery saved many dollars. Savings to a hospital are impressive when considering the cost of replacing a single nurse (Hoffman, 1985). Other savings in indirect costs, such as decreased accidents and illnesses, fewer sick days, and averted lawsuits and complaints are not as easy to document (Sullivan, 1986). However, it is not easy to acquire adequate funding to ensure that chemical dependency problems are interrupted and treated in a timely manner.

The work of most state nursing associations' peer assistance programs is still conducted predominantly on a volunteer basis. Volunteers have only limited time. Some state nurses' associations have little or no funds designated for the programs, although some staff time, or mailing and telephone back-up might be allocated.

The costs of treatment services are usually borne by a third-party payer (insurance companies or Medicare) or by the nurse in treatment. Most third-party payers cover chemical dependency treatment, although the length of stay covered for inpatient care has been shortened and coverage may be limited to one particular program. Some states require medical insurance companies to offer optional coverage. Many people reject the offer, thinking they would never need it. A few states require coverage. Residential (inpatient) treatment is more likely to be covered than outpatient care and hospitals more likely than free-standing facilities even though the latter are equally effective and less expensive. Follow-up continuing care may or may not be covered by insurance, although it is sometimes included as part of a residential treatment "package." Some private providers of chemical dependency treatment, such as psychologists and licensed counselors, may be eligible for third-party reimbursement, but few nurses in private practice with chemically dependent clients have been able to secure third-party payment for their services.

It is obvious that many nurses do not have funding sources for treatment and, thus are not receiving sufficient help. They may, of course, recover through AA and NA, but successful maintenance of sobriety through mutual support group assistance alone requires a great deal of self-awareness and self-motivation that many nurses have not achieved. Treatment helps penetrate denial and allows the nurse to learn healthy coping skills, prepare for lifestyle changes, and plan for the future, all within a relatively short period. Without treatment, successful rehabilitation can take many years.

CHAPTER 8

DISCIPLINARY ACTION AND REGULATORY BOARDS

The preceding chapters have explained how competent, well-planned intervention, treatment, and job reentry programs can improve a chemically dependent nurse's prospects for recovery and return to work. However, relapses, failed recovery, and refusal to accept treatment will still occur. To protect public safety, it is important to maintain disciplinary and regulatory systems that ensure that chemically dependent nurses do not jeopardize patient safety. The chemically dependent nurse needs to know that his or her professional future is at stake. There are circumstances that necessitate job reassignment, firing, and even revocation of the nurse's license.

WHEN TO RESORT TO DISCIPLINARY ACTION

Institution of disciplinary action against a chemically dependent nurse *should* be a difficult judgment call, if we are to avoid the "throwaway nurse syndrome," in which the problem is "solved" by firing the nurse and/or revoking the nursing license. Disciplinary action may jeopardize the nurse's income, career path, family life, and personal sense of well-being. The decision to institute disciplinary action should be carefully considered.

If the firing of a nurse is not reported to the state board of nursing, public safety will still be endangered. The nurse may be able to find employment at another institution or in another state. Too often, the addicted nurse is encouraged by the employer to leave and find employment elsewhere. If nurses are indeed guilty of misappropriating controlled substances or working while intoxicated, they hesitate to resist the employer's actions for fear of exposure and embarrassment. The nurse is given a lukewarm, but not blatantly negative, reference and the employer escapes potential litigation, but the real problem is transferred to the new employer. If the problem warrants dismissal, it likely warrants the attention of the state board of nursing.

Mandatory Reporting

Some states have passed legislation, the so-called "snitch laws," that require observers to report drug-abusing nurses to the board of nursing. In some states this requirement is limited to cases in which a nurse is practicing while impaired; in other states, however, the law requires the reporting of all drug use incidents, whether or not addiction is present. The mandatory reporting requirement may be included in the state's nursing practice act, or in supplemental legislation. For example, some states, in an attempt to confront malpractice considerations, have enacted tort reform legislation that includes a required reporting provision. While these mandatory reporting laws are rarely enforced, they do open the door to civil liability if a patient is hurt. These laws may have encouraged employers to obscure the real reasons for the firing or reassignment of a chemically dependent nurse to cover their negligence in reporting to the board of nursing. On the other hand, these laws have probably encouraged some health care professionals to take more seriously their own responsibilities in protecting the public.

When to Report

Hospitals vary in their policies on reporting a nurse to the state board of nursing. Patient safety must be the primary criterion for reporting.

Are patients being placed in jeopardy by the continued practice of a nurse who is actively abusing alcohol or other drugs? If the nurse is not placing patients in danger and is attempting to confront the illness in an employer or peer assistance program, the report may be deferred and may eventually prove unnecessary. A report should include information about the people involved, the dates and times, what was observed and by who, and reference to any available documentation. This information should be gathered and retained even if the report is held pending the nurse's satisfactory participation in an employer or peer assistance program. Should the nurse's participation be unsatisfactory, the necessary documentation will be available.

In summary, a report to the state board of nursing is not a diagnosis of addiction per se; it is a factual report of specific events. The purpose of the report is not to prove a nurse's violation of the nurse practice act, but rather to provide a well-documented record of actions and events.

THE BOARD OF NURSING

Although some states' nursing boards encourage and participate in intervention programs, their primary responsibility is to ensure public safety. They are licensing boards, charged not only with determining licensure suitability, but also with meting out sanctions for violations.

Legal Constraints

In most states the nursing board's legislative mandate is the nurse practice act, which specifies the conditions under which a license is granted, revoked or withheld. It also outlines additional options under which the board may issue summary suspensions, voluntary surrender of license, and other forms of licensure restriction.

The board must work with the state's attorney general to enforce the law. Boards are usually reactive, limiting their activities to cases that are reported to them. They do not engage in case-finding. State boards handle more cases of narcotics use than any of other drugs of dependency, including alcohol, marijuana, cocaine, and benzodiazapines. This is because most cases are reported to the board only when there is a clear, documented infringement of the law. Cases are presented after an appointed investigator has discovered enough sub-stantial evidence to support the charges. When narcotics have been stolen from a hospital or records falsified, there is a case for practice act violations. Use of illegal"street drugs" is more difficult to prove, es-pecially if they are not used at the workplace (even if impaired job performance is observed). With alleged abuse of alcohol and pre-scription drugs, particularly if the latter are prescribed by a physician, excessive use and patient risk must be proved. Unless the nurse is discovered intoxicated on duty and the event solidly documented at that time, the violation may be difficult to demonstrate.

Political Constraints

Most state nursing boards consist of political appointees, some of who are lay members and many of who may be unfamiliar with the nature of addictive illness and methods of rehabilitation. Their decisions may be motivated by a desire to avoid controversy and risk rather than by an enlightened understanding of the value and benefits of rehabilitation. For example, when a long-sober, recovered alcoholic nurse from another state applied for a license to one state nursing board, she was candid about her history, including her ongoing AA membership. She was refused the license on the grounds that she had not yet conquered her problem, as evidenced by her own admission that she continued to attend AA meetings. The services of an attorney were required to resolve this matter. Appendix H contains tables of licensure violations and disciplinary actions taken by state boards of nursing in 1985.

Institution of more effective education about chemical dependency may reduce misinformed judgment like the one above, but state boards are likely to maintain a conservative stance in reviewing licensure of the chemically dependent nurse. Again, the board's priority is patient safety, and flexibility and trust in the nurse could put the public at risk. As a disciplinary body for chemical dependency problems and for many other kinds of professional misconduct, board members are subjected to endless excuses and numerous lies. They observe the downside of the nursing profession year after year. It is not surprising that they sometimes become skeptical and concentrate their efforts on weeding out rather than retrieving the offending nurses.

Roles and Responsibilities

Many state boards *do* take a strong interest in rehabilitation, however, their formal role in such efforts may be limited. The Missouri State Board of nursing, for instance, appointed a task force in 1984 to review the issue and make recommendations. The peer assistance program of the Missouri Nurses' Association was formed as a result of this task force. This Missouri State Board of Nursing continues to demonstrate their interest in the individual nurse while continuing to protect the public. This attitude is illustrated by the following statement from Florence McGuire, Executive Director of the Missouri State Board of Nursing, which appeared in the March 1987 issue of the board's *Newsletter* (pp. 2–3).

The primary purpose of occupational licensing laws is to protect the health and welfare of the public. The Board of Nursing was created by law at the insistence of the profession and the public that safe nursing care be assured. The State Board of Nursing utilizes three methods of regulation to accomplish this fact:
1.   Setting standards and granting approval for schools of nursing.
2.   Determining eligibility for initial licensure and relicensure.
3.   Taking disciplinary action against licensed individuals who violate the Nursing Practice Act.

The types of disciplinary action available to the Board by law are censure, probation, suspension, revocation and any combination of the above. Censure is the least restrictive form and is simply a letter issued by the Board for violation of the law. It will state the specific behavior which has caused the Board to be concerned. A copy is placed in the individual's record and retained permanently. Probation requires that the nurse meet certain terms established by the Board. Terms may include counseling, letters of evaluation from employers, etc. Probation may not exceed five (5) years and the nurse still retains licensure with the ability to work. Suspension means that the nurse is prohibited from practice for a specified period of time not to exceed three (3) years. Licensure is removed from the individual during that period of time. Upon completion of the period of suspension the license may be returned to the individual. Revocation is the severest form of discipline. The license is taken away and may be obtained only after the same qualifications as for initial licensure are met. That requires permission being granted by the Board to sit for NCLEX and subsequently passing with acceptable scores.

Frequently the Board may utilize a combination of any of the four (4) actions previously mentioned. The most common combination is to order a harsh discipline such as revocation then stay that order and issue a lessor discipline such as probation.

The number of disciplinary actions taken by the Board has risen from four (4) in 1981 to fifty-eight (58) in 1986. Of those disciplined in 1986 86% to 90% were chemical abuse related. The drastic increase in numbers has been of great concern to the Board and in August of 1984 they convened the first meeting of the Impaired Nurse Task Force to grapple with the increasing problem of chemical abuse among nurses.

The Task Force presented recommendations to the Board of Nursing and the Board subsequently requested the Missouri Nurses' Association to establish and maintain a Peer Assistance Program.

Due to the concern of the individual members of the Board of Nursing for their impaired peers along with mandated concern as a regulatory agency for the clients who are served by those nurses, disciplining with the necessary follow-up has become a very heavy load. Every Board Meeting lasts four (4) to five (5) days with two (2) to three (3) days being almost entirely devoted to some segment of the disciplinary process whether it be consideration of investigative reports, disciplinary hearings, probationary meetings or hearings for violation of probation. The Board of Nursing is most eager to have a successfully functioning Peer Assistance Program in place for the benefit of all.

Because of concern for their peers as individuals and the inherent need of nurses to help others, the Board of Nursing views the MoNA-PRN (Missouri Nurses' Association—Project Recovering Nurse) Program as the approach that is preferred for dealing with nurses with impaired practice. It would seem to be a much more practical and effective approach, in some instances, to give assistance to an impaired individual through a system of confrontation, evaluation, treatment and follow-up that also includes continued monitoring and support by one's peers than to take the more punitive approach allowed for in the law.

Through participation on the Peer Assistance Committee which was established by MoNA (Missouri Nurses' Association), the Board has had continuous input into the MoNA-PRN Program. Progress has been reported periodically to the Board by the Committee in regard to the established process. The Board continues to be mindful of the legislative mandate to guard the safety of the public and takes that charge very seriously while at the same time, trying to establish a means more considerate of the problems of the individual nurses involved. Because of close cooperation between MoNA and the Board of Nursing, a nurse may be in the MoNA-PRN Program without first being reported to the Board or, on the other hand, an impaired nurse may be referred to the PRN Program after first being reported to the Board but prior to the necessary discipline which might have been taken on the license. If the individual does not stay in compliance with the requirements of the PRN Program she/he will then be reported to the Board of Nursing for discipline.

In June, 1986, when MoNA-PRN requested permission to commence the Pilot Project, the Board was monitoring around fifty (50) people who had been placed on probation or given a period of suspension followed by probation. In the past all who were placed on suspension or probation were requested to appear for a meeting with the Board at which time they were expected to show evidence of working toward recovery/rehabilitation. The Board has felt that evidence is best demonstrated through evaluations from employers and counselors, signed attendance at AA/NA meetings or other support groups, and other requirements which may be unique to the individual situation. Some nurses may elect to continue to be monitored by the Board but many may choose to be monitored by MoNA-PRN when given that alternative.

Board Actions

State boards commonly respond to a nurse's impaired practice due to alcohol or other drugs in one of three ways:

1. They may refuse to restore or grant a license.

2. They may rely on a host of experts to testify about whether the nurse's addiction poses a hazard, thus providing some degree of assurance of patient safety as well as someone with whom to share the responsibility if the nurse fails.

3. They may institute or cooperate with a strict and thorough monitoring system designed to discover relapse. Strict monitoring is expensive and intrusive, but it can reduce the public's risk to an acceptable level.

A state board is rarely severely criticized for being excessively cautious or conservative, however, it may be mercilessly attacked if a nurse it has permitted to practice harms a patient while chemically impaired.

Some state boards have found ways to protect public safety *and* rehabilitate impaired nurses with "diversion" legislation described in Chapter 7. Because the majority of states have not developed such legislation, the National Nurses Society on Addictions issued a *Statement on Model Diversion Legislation for Chemically Impaired Nurses* in 1984, the text of which can be found in Appendix F. The statement, written by one of these authors (EW), provides a model for other states to follow or adapt as they begin to develop diversion legislation. The model strives to provide protection for the public (patients), the impaired nurse, the nurse's employer, the nurse's supervisors, and for those involved in EAPs and/or peer assistance efforts.

The model allows the board of nursing to work with an EAP or with the state nursing association's peer assistance program. All programs, however, must reflect accepted principles of treatment, monitoring, and confidentiality. The model also covers such issues as the suggested expunging of records of nurses who have sustained recovery without relapse for five years.

If a nurse is referred to the board after unsuccessful recovery efforts, the model legislation can provide the means to document the violation of the practice act.

The model empowers the state regulatory agency as a strong advocate of the diversion procedure. Most regulatory bodies will welcome this change in the nurse practice act when it is clear that it will provide better protection for the public through a structured system of identification, intervention, treatment, and monitoring.

CHAPTER 9

DRUG TESTING

Considerable controversy surrounds the usefulness, accuracy, and legality of the use of laboratory urinalysis to test for drug use. Urinalyses reports can indicate the presence of drugs when none were used and, conversely, yield a negative report when drugs have indeed been used. According to *U.S. News & World Report* (July 28, 1986), "The most common test has a 1-in-20 rate of false positives" (p. 51). Furthermore, drug testing can verify one's use of a drug but cannot demonstrate chemical dependency.

In addition, the legal right to test for drugs without one's consent is controversial. This chapter will discuss drug testing procedures, definitions, the chance of error, and the ethical and legal issues involved.

DRUG TESTING MEASUREMENTS

Drugs may be taken orally, rectally, or nasally. They may also be injected into muscle or vein, smoked, or absorbed by the skin. Drugs are carried by blood to the liver where they are metabolized and released back into the bloodstream as metabolites. Metabolites and unchanged drugs are detectable in body fluids (blood and urine) and gases (breath). The presence of a drug's metabolite in blood, urine, breath, or hair may be considered evidence of use. Because most drug screening in the workplace is by urinalysis, we will focus on that procedure.

Urinalysis reveals drug metabolites as they are being excreted from the body in urine. Drug excretion rates vary from less than one hour to several months. One study of 86 men in a controlled, abstinent environment revealed the presence of marijuana in their urine for 77 days after their last use (Ellis, Mann, Judson, Schramm, & Tashcian, 1985). Chlordiazapoxide (Librium®) is excreted in about one week, alcohol in less than 24 hours.

Drug tests provide a limited estimate of a user's degree of impairment because they reveal only the drug's presence in the recent past. Impairment may occur as a withdrawal syndrome after the drug has been cleared from the body. Except during early withdrawal, tests would, of course, be negative. Table 9–1 shows the length of time some types of drugs remain in the body.

Table 9-1 Drug Detection Period

DRUG	TYPE	DETECTION PERIOD
amphetamine	stimulant	2–4 days
barbiturate	sedative	12 hours–3 weeks
cocaine	stimulant	2–4 days
fentanyl	narcotic analgesic	can be less than an hour
heroin/morphine/ meperidine (Demerol)	narcotic analgesic	2–4 days
marijuana	euphoric	3 days–more than one month
methadone	analgesic	2–4 days
PCP	anesthetic	1-30 days
benzodiazepine	tranquilizer	up to 1 week

Definitions

The following definitions will help clarify the drug-testing process.

Sensitivity The detection limit of the test. The more sensitive the test, the longer the drug can be detected and the smaller the amount that can be measured; also the greater the risk of "false positives."

Specificity The ability of a test to discriminate between drugs. The more specific the test, the more accurate the determination of specific drug use.

False Results The erroneous reporting of drug presence. Results are reported as negative or positive and determined by a cut-off point on the concentration measurement scale. Results can be reported erroneously for reasons such as contamination of the urine specimen or the container, ingestion of certain foods, body weight, the amount of liquids consumed, over-the-counter or other medications taken, the

Table 9-2 Substances Interfering with Drug Test Results

BRAND NAME	INTERFERES WITH	MIMICS	TIME
Vicks Formula 44-M Triaminic DM	immunoassay	opiates	1 day
Primatene	immunoassay MS/GC	barbiturates	13 days
Dietac Dexatrim Cotylenol Triaminic	immunoassay	amphetamines	1 day
Benadryl	immunoassay	methadone	1–2 days
Primatene Bronkotabs Nyquil	immunoassay	amphetamines	1–2 days
Midol Premensin Primatene-M	immunoassay	opiates	no data

type of test used, and the quality of the laboratory and technicians performing the analysis. Human error is a common cause of false results.

False Positive An erroneous result indicating the false presence of a drug. A false positive usually occurs when a harmless substance (eg poppy seeds) causes the same reaction as an addictive drug (eg opiates) and is reported as drug positive. Table 9-2 identifies common over-the-counter medications that cause false positive results.

False Negative An erroneous result indicating the absence of a drug that actually is present. A false negative is reported if the the drug is not present in high enough concentration to exceed the cut-off point. False negatives can result when copious amounts of liquids have been consumed or when the cut-off point is too high to be sufficiently sensitive to the quantity of drug present.

Assay The analysis of a substance to determine its composition.

Screening Assay An analysis used to screen a sample for the presence of drugs. Samples testing positive with a screening assay should be followed by a confirmation assay to ensure that the result is not false positive.

Confirmation Assay A follow-up test, more sensitive and more specific than the screening test, to confirm the presence of a drug. When the presence of drugs is not validated by the confirmation assay, the test is reported as negative.

Cross-Reactivity The misidentification of a drug when the reaction of one metabolite mimics the presence of another. For example, novocaine can be reported as cocaine.

Nanograms and Micrograms Concentrations of metabolites in urine that are reported as amounts per milliliter. The amounts are reported as nanograms (ng) or micrograms (µg). There are 1,000 nanograms in one microgram. A microgram is one-millionth of one gram. There are 28 million micrograms in one ounce. The presence of marijuana is usually reported in nanograms per milliliter, while cocaine metabolite is reported in micrograms per milliliter.

Quality Assurance (QA) The ability of a laboratory to conduct consistently accurate tests. To meet high-quality assurance standards, rigorously controlled procedures should be followed in handling, storing, labeling, and testing samples for the presence of drugs. To test a laboratory for QA, a nursing administrator can send urine containing a known quantity of a drug. The laboratory's ability to produce accurate results can be determined by comparing its report with the known quantity. The known samples are referred to as quality control samples.

No test is absolutely accurate. The chance, however, that drug users will test negative is greater than the chance that non-drug users will test positive. When proper precautions are taken and a urinalysis is positive for drugs, one can be fairly certain that the results are accurate. Sometimes specimens are split and some of the original is retained until the report is received. Positive reports can then be verified by testing a second time before the result is accepted.

DRUG TESTS AND PROCEDURES

Thin Layer Chromatography (TLC)

TLC is commonly used to detect very high recent doses of drugs or toxic levels of drugs. It is extremely useful in emergency room admissions for drug overdose cases in which a patient is unable to report what or how much of a drug has been taken. However, the test is not sensitive enough to use in drug screens in the workplace since only very large doses are detected. False negatives are common for people using smaller quantities.

Gas Chromatography (GC) and Gas Chromatograph Mass Spectrometer (GC-MS)

Gas chromatography and gas chromatography mass spectrometer is about 100 to 1,000 times more sensitive than TLC; it will also specifically identify the drugs present. A urine sample is heated to a vapor inside a gas chromatogram, which measures the amount of time the vaporized drug takes to pass through a column filled with testing substances. This test can identify extremely small quantities of several drugs in a single analysis. Its sensitivity can be increased with mass spectrometry, which breaks down drug vapor into smaller fragments that are measured for electrical charge. Although these tests are considered the most reliable, they are also expensive, time-consuming, and require complex procedures. With the increased computerization of laboratories, however, these tests are becoming more widely used.

Enzyme Immunoassay (EIA) and Radioimmunoassay (RIA)

Enzyme immunoassay and radioimmunoassay use the sensitivity and specificity of antibodies to indicate the type and quantity of drug metabolites present in the urine. For EIA, the urine sample is mixed with reagents used to detect specific drugs. The mixture is placed in a spectrometer, which measures the amount of light the mixture

Table 9-3 Comparison of Laboratory Tests for Drug Screening

NAME	TYPE	SENSITIVITY	SPECIFICITY	AVAILABILITY
TLC	toxicology screen	poor	poor	inexpensive, fast, can be done in most labs
GC GC-MS	chemical analysis	excellent	excellent	expensive, requires complex equipment and trained personnel, available in some labs
RIA EIA	immunoassay	excellent	good	moderate cost, available in many labs, easily automated procedures

absorbs. The degree of absorption indicates the presence or absence of the drug. RIA uses radioactive substances similarly.

Sometimes cross-reaction of compounds can occur, making RIA and EIA less specific than GC or GC-MS. Nevertheless, RIA and EIA are commonly used for screening assays because the laboratory procedure is less complex, more widely available, and less expensive.

Table 9-3 compares the various tests for drug screening.

SOURCES OF INACCURATE RESULTS

Interference, deliberate or accidental, in the drug testing procedure can occur at any step in the process and may cause results to be reported incorrectly.

Collecting the Specimen

Ideally the specimen should be a supervised, first-void urine, but any specimen collected entirely unannounced and closely supervised can be used. It is essential that the container be clean and remain uncontaminated with any substance. In addition, the specimen should be transported and stored at room temperature or cooler because heat can destroy drug metabolites and result in a false negative report.

Other Medications

As previously stated, a false positive can result when certain over-the-counter medications or foods are taken. Table 9-2 gives examples of brand-name cold, allergy, and pain medications that interfere with the accuracy of urinalysis drug tests. These and other medications may erroneously suggest the presence of mood-altering chemicals.

Laboratory Quality Control

Inaccurate results can occur with poorly trained personnel or ill-equipped laboratories. With the recent popularity of urinalysis for drug screening, many laboratories have added or increased their capabilities for these tests. It is important to determine the adequacy and accuracy of their procedures, especially when careers and reputations depend on the results.

A laboratory can be selected after a quality assurance check. The laboratory should report positive or negative results as well as the actual quantity of drug metabolite present.

Deliberate Sabotage

Despite precautions, test results can be altered by various methods. Some of these methods include:

O Placing various chemical substances under the fingernails to release into the sample

O Puncturing the specimen container with a pin thus allowing the urine to escape slowly during transport

O Adding soap from restroom dispensers to the specimen

O Releasing fluid from a fluid-filled bulb (placed under the arm with a tube leading to the genitalia) into the container in place of urine

O Procuring urine from drug-free friends or saving own urine from non-drug use periods and substituting it for newly voided specimen

O Scooping water from the commode to dilute the specimen

O Concealing plastic tube filled with drug-free urine in vagina, unscrewing cap, and "urinating" into container

O Sending friend to give specimen

O Catheterizing own bladder and substituting urine obtained from a family member, then urinating under careful observation

There are many ways to outwit urine collectors, and the chance that a positive result is accurate is far more likely than belief in erroneous negative findings.

ETHICAL AND LEGAL ISSUES IN TESTING

The ethical and legal issues concerning use of drug testing to monitor a recovering nurse have been discussed in Chapter 6. There is a significant difference between testing known and suspected nurses and random tests of whole populations. Yet some argue that there are certain occupations in which drug impaired performance is potentially so dangerous to the welfare of others that careful investigation and screening of their members is essential. (This argument has been applied to professions ranging from airline pilots to baseball players.) A comprehensive discussion of the constitutional, legal, and ethical issues related to random drug screening is beyond the scope of this book, but we believe that it is a very real and pressing concern to the nursing profession. Reasonable concern for patient safety requires that a recovering nurse be closely monitored for any indication of relapse. Because careful attention to the procedures of specimen collection and laboratory analysis can reduce the chance of error, random drug screens do provide the best guarantee that the nurse is remaining drug-free.

Responsible Handling of Drug Testing

While debate on the larger issues of random drug screening continues, the following general conditions are proposed as guidelines for responsible handling of drug testing for chemically dependent nurses:

1. Drug testing should be reserved for nurses whose job performance indicates an addiction problem.

2. Drug testing should be done carefully and thoroughly, with affirmation of laboratory quality assurance.

3. When drug testing is part of the monitoring of a recovering nurse, there should be a scheduled review of the status and progress, and testing should be discontinued when no longer appropriate.

4. Disclosure of test results should be limited to "need to know" staff.

5. Specimens should be tested for alcohol and other drugs, not for any other condition. (Specimens can reveal pregnancy and the presence of unrelated diseases.)

The current widespread debates about drug testing are not yet concluded, however, it is prudent to inform employees of drug testing policies and procedures and the latter should be reasonable and protective of the legal rights of employees.

CHAPTER 10

ETHICAL CONSIDERATIONS

To qualify as a profession, an occupational group is expected to possess a specialized body of knowledge, a concern for its peers, and a code of ethics. (See Appendix I for American Nurses' Association Code for Nurses.) A professional group may also claim the authority to determine the specific knowledge, skills, and attributes its members must possess. Outsiders may be included as advisors in this process, but professionals believe that they best understand the nature of their work.

A professional group must also assume responsibility for its standards. Self-regulation of professional standards can be difficult and unpleasant, and most professional groups experience a constant state of tension. They must balance a commitment to standards of professional conduct against the natural reluctance to expose awkward and embarrassing situations among their colleagues.

In the nursing profession, there is no disagreement that the primary responsibility is to protect patients from the adverse consequences of a nurse's chemical dependency. Nor is there significant disagreement on the need to identify chemically dependent nurses and to help them prevent damage to themselves and avoid the loss of their talents to the profession. The debate concerns the methods of achieving these goals. The choices have serious consequences and raise many ethical questions.

Coercion

Chemical dependency management must address the powerful denial that is characteristic of the disease, as well as the specific organic damage that can affect treatment outcome. Alcohol and other drugs affect the ability to think, reason, feel, and act, so decisions about appropriate treatment cannot be left to the chemically dependent nurse.

Denial is such a central factor in this disease that often the chemically dependent nurse sincerely does not believe the existence of a dependency situation. There may be emotional problems, "blackouts," or even periods of total amnesia due to the organic effects of alcohol and other drugs that confuse perceptions of reality. In this situation, colleagues must coerce a nurse into a treatment situation that is not likely to be voluntarily accepted. There may be tears, anger, and appeals that family and financial obligations will be neglected during treatment. The intervenor must resist the temptation to compromise and must deal with the discomfort of forcing agreement to unwanted treatment.

Many residential treatment centers do not accept patients whose admission is ordered under formal commitment procedures. "Voluntary" admission is required, and in a strictly legal sense, it *is* voluntary. In reality, most patients enter chemical-dependency treatment under a strong form of coercion. Some are threatened with loss of custody of children; others with divorce; some are offered treatment as an alternative to jail; others face job or license loss.

False Accusations

Although coercion is often necessary, it also creates the potential for abuse. Because denial is so strong, diagnosis of this disease must come from the observations and reports of others. Such interventions are usually the result of genuine concern and desire to interrupt the progress of the disease; however, there is also the possibility of false accusation. There is a great deal at stake—the welfare of patients, the financial health and public image of the hospital, as well as the health and personal welfare of the nurse.

If treatment must be coerced, certain guidelines, including careful, accurate documentation of a problem, should be followed. Rare though it is, people who were not addicts have been sent to addiction-specific treatment. With denial so prevalent, the protests of a genuinely innocent person may be disbelieved.

Intervention must be firm and uncompromising, but it need never be brutal. The goal is to steer a sick person incapable of good judgment into a safe situation in which the effects of the drugs can be cleared. Eventually, when the ability to reason returns, the person regains the ability to make choices. This takes time and structure and others may have to temporarily take charge of the person's life.

In assuming responsibility for another person, the most important decision the caretaker will make is the choice of a treatment program. The well-being of the patient should be the primary consideration during program choice. Conflict of interest should be avoided in referral situations. Only in unusual circumstances should a nurse undergo treatment at his or her workplace.

GUILT AND SHAME

If we adopt the attitude that chemical dependency is a disease and not a matter of choice, we must confront the issues of personal responsibility and blame. There are those who fear that if the chemically dependent nurse is not to be considered responsible for becoming an addict, then the damaging behavior may continue while others take responsibility for paying the bills and repairing the damage. The classification of addiction as a disease does not, however, absolve the ill person from responsibility for undergoing treatment and maintaining recovery.

The addict does not choose addiction, just as the diabetic does not choose diabetes. The diabetic cannot be expected to invent a proper diet or discover insulin, but can indeed be expected to exercise, lose weight, follow a proper diet and health care regimen, and take the appropriate medication. Likewise, the alcoholic or other drug addict, when appropriately treated and rehabilitated, can be held partially responsible for the outcome.

After recovery, however, ethical dilemmas remain. Despite their powerful efforts to make amends, some chemically dependent nurses may still be faced with irretrievable personal losses. The clock cannot be turned back. There will be promotions missed, courses not taken, articles only half-read or poorly comprehended. There may be memories of successfully concealed mistakes. When a physician was asked if she had ever harmed a patient during her active addiction, she replied, "I must have, I could only read about half of my records." A man in nursing told of dropping the tip of a catheter but sending it for culture anyway, rather than admit to clumsiness. It happened years ago, but he still feels shame.

Perhaps nurses, and others for whom idealism was a significant aspect of their career choice, experience a heightened sense of guilt and pain for their failures. Violation of one's ethical standards can be the greatest torment during the recovery process. Guilt can, however, be an asset when it helps reinforce the determination to recover and avoid relapse. Most nurses in recovery have no need of additional punishment.

CHAPTER 11

LOOKING TO THE FUTURE: RECOMMENDATIONS FOR CHANGE

There is a popular cartoon in which a couple is sitting in a living room, entertaining guests. Behind the sofa stands an enormous, frightening-looking animal. The captions reads: "We deal with it by not talking about it."

Along with other professions, the nursing profession has indeed begun to talk about "it." A recent exchange in a major nursing journal, however, indicates that disagreement remains. An editorial pleaded with the nursing profession to stop publicizing its members' problems with drug abuse (Kelly, 1986). Letters of reply were equally strong in urging that the openness continue (Naegle, 1987).

The nursing profession must continue to examine this problem openly and to engage in energetic debate of the best solution. In addition, we must augment our data base with careful research findings. We must enhance the nursing education curricula to overcome the continuing and unacceptable ignorance of the deadly disease. And beyond enhancing our knowledge of chemical dependency, we must discover better methods of assistance for nurses who suffer from it.

Research

Little research has been done on chemical dependency among nurses. The authors of this book are among the pioneers in pursuing these studies. Bissell is the first researcher to study a large sample (N = 100) of nurses from the national population (Bissell & Jones, 1981). Her work included a five- to seven-year follow-up of the nurses in the original study (Bissell & Haberman, 1984). Sullivan (1987) surveyed a national population of both dependent (N = 139) and nondependent (N = 384) nurses. Others (Brennan, 1983; Kelley, 1985; Hutchinson, 1986; Reed, 1986) have studied smaller samples of recovered chemically dependent nurses. Wood (1985) surveyed a large nationwide sample (N = 1,134) of registered nurses for concerns about their own and colleagues' drinking or drug-taking behaviors. These descriptive studies have contributed to our comprehension of the complexity and diversity of the chemically dependent population, however many questions remain.

Epidemiology

We do not have a satisfactory estimate of the number of nurses with alcohol or drug problems. Nor have we documented the causes of dependency or determined the best means of recovery assistance. How do we establish what is the most desirable treatment and who should provide it? How is success measured? We have only clinical impressions and anecdotal accounts to guide us. Are there characteristics about nurses or nursing that make dependency more likely? Which characteristics are relevant to recovery? Do environmental variables, such as employer support, licensure sanctions, and family members' participation in recovery programs, assist with recovery or mitigate it?

A handful of good research papers have appeared, however, most of the important questions about chemical dependency in nursing remain unanswered. Because we do not know how many nurses are now or have been affected, it is impossible to know whether matters are improving or deteriorating. We lack the baseline against which to measure. Description of subpopulations, such as those whose licenses were revoked or those seen at a particular treatment facility, do not provide sound estimates of the prevalence of the disease. We need basic epidemiologic studies to reveal how many nurses are involved, then we can begin to describe trends and evaluate whether we are gaining or losing ground.

Research Issues

In addition, we have not adequately studied the nursing profession itself. Does nursing attract potentially chemically dependent people? Does the practice of nursing contribute to a greater or lesser likelihood that one will develop the disease? We offer anecdotal evidence to answer these questions, but we do not know if we can generalize these data to the larger population of chemically dependent nurses. We will not know until careful studies have been designed and implemented.

In a world of diversity, we must not assume that all nurses are the same. Studies evaluating important cultural differences must include and differentiate between men and women, minorities, non-Americans, and other subgroups.

The populations seen by disciplinary boards and those seen only by treatment centers, mutual help, or nurses' support groups are probably quite different. This is not surprising, since they are at different stages of illness and are addicted to different drugs. Disciplinary boards are more likely to follow the more advanced cases or those whose drugs are detectably diverted from the workplace.

Other questions must be addressed. Is one treatment system better than another? How long should a nurse be monitored? When can the nurse safely return to work and under what conditions? Are there high-risk clinical areas? If so, do particular types of people seek them out or do the settings themselves contribute to the problem? Are settings chosen because drugs are freely available or supervision casual? Do circumstances on a particular unit make it easier to start using drugs?

Addictive illnesses could be approached like progressive illnesses such as cancer, which if ignored and allowed to persist, will predictably worsen. We can then examine the age at which a nurse becomes "clean" (free of non-alcoholic drugs) or "dry" (free of alcohol) and the total time lapsed between the onset of drug/alcohol use and total recovery. The achievement of abstinence at a younger age or after fewer years of total drug use might be perceived as positive and we could attempt to identify the actions or circumstances leading to early abstinence.

Prevention Research

Prevention research, although difficult, is not impossible and is definitely necessary. First we have to decide exactly what we hope to prevent and then be willing to test our efforts. It may be possible to prevent first use of a drug or to instill an ethic that would forbid the offering of mood-altering drugs to a colleague. Once a drug has been tried and found rewarding, it is much harder to use in moderation.

Attempts to prevent young peoples' first use of tobacco have been somewhat successful; it may also be possible for nurses to avoid initial and hence subsequent drug involvements. Drug-use attitudes and decisions may, however, be established before nursing school. It may also be possible to convince nurses that certain drugs are never, under any circumstances, to be self-prescribed.

To address the many pressing questions about chemical dependency among nurses and to develop further the knowledge base begun by early researchers, a cadre of research-prepared nurses and other scientists must be established. The education of nurse researchers is still in its infancy. These scientists ideally should have research preparation at the doctoral level. They should collaborate with skilled researchers in nursing as well as with researchers in other disciplines (medicine, psychology, social work, sociology). No area of knowledge should be ignored.

With the passage of Congressional legislation in 1985 establishing the National Center for Nursing Research (NCNR) within the National Institutes of Health (NIH), nursing is gaining credibility as a discipline whose problems are worthy of scientific study. The NCNR's funding priorities focus on problems that impact patient care; research to reduce chemical dependency among nurses would certainly help protect patients.

MANDATE FOR EDUCATION

Nurses who have become addicted to alcohol and other drugs believe that their schooling left them unprepared to recognize the dangers of drug or alcohol dependency or to understand its signs and symptoms. The basic lack of information slowed their awareness and made it harder for them to accept their illness (or that of a colleague or family member) when others finally attempted to confront them.

We recommend that a massive and comprehensive education program be mounted in the nursing profession for the benefit of nurses, their families, and their patients. A model curriculum is provided in Appendix A. We believe that schools of nursing (graduate and undergraduate), employers of nurses, and boards of nursing must work together to develop course content requirements for student nurses and practicing nurses. There are almost 2 million nurses in the country today, but few of them are educated or experienced in this field. They care for chemically dependent clients, they have colleagues who have or may develop the disease, and they are at risk for it themselves. Most people in all three categories will die from the disease if it remains unrecognized and untreated. We believe that protection of the public and of nurses is necessary and requires an immediate and comprehensive educational program.

Most professional schools still fail to distinguish between the toxic effects of alcohol and other drugs on different body systems, their pharmacology, and the addictive illness itself. Even physical dependency and the more subtle effects of withdrawal are given little attention in most curricula.

Nurses must learn about the disease, including signs and symptoms of early problems as well as strategies for intervention and assistance. They must learn to recognize that risk is widespread, and that there are many early warning signs that must be taken seriously when noted in themselves and in colleagues. They must also realize that effective treatment is available if carefully sought and that the legality and availability of a drug reveals little about its dangers. Alcohol continues to kill many more of its users than do narcotics and it causes a more serious form of physical dependency. Death during withdrawal from alcohol is common, whereas it is quite rare with narcotics or cocaine.

Even the common physical signs of sedative drug dependence are poorly covered in most curricula. Alcohol is the most common underlying cause of "essential" hypertension and of mild adult-onset diabetes. Alone or in combination with the minor tranquilizers or soporifics, it accounts for most "idiopathic" adult-onset grand mal seizures. Most alcoholism treatment services are accustomed to patients with histories of unmonitored treatment with Dilantin® antihypertensives, and oral hypogycemics. Mild tachycardia, mild intention tremors, slightly elevated temperatures, fluid retention (three or four pounds that vanish on the third or fourth hospital day) are all indications of heavy use of alcohol.

Many health care professionals are not aware that withdrawal of alcohol and other sedatives often causes insomnia as well as agitated depression. When these signs appear, a tense and nervous person may assume he or she needs minor tranquilizers and so drinks alcohol instead. Symptoms may be easily overlooked or misinterpreted if one is accustomed to considering only extreme withdrawal states or of the injection of opiates as signs of addiction. Once the cart is firmly placed before the horse, it is easy to understand why reports of marital discord, accidents, mood swings at work, and a host of other signals that might alert the nurse or her colleagues are also misunderstood.

Nursing education, therefore, must include better basic information for students as well as faculty. It should include material on all psychotropic drugs, licit and illicit (prescription drugs can also be addictive and misused), liquid, solid, smoked, injected, or inhaled. We must concentrate on the effects of chemical dependency, not on the legality of particular drugs. Just as alcohol has been legal and illegal at varying times and places in our nation's history, so too have cocaine and the opiates. The decisions about legality and distribution are made, after all, by people and often do not reflect the real degree of danger a drug may pose.

Nursing students and faculty are not alone in their educational needs; the majority of people in health care now rely on continuing education courses and journals to stay current or to make up for past deficits. Addictive illness is so common and already of such national concern that methods must be developed to educate a larger proportion of people in the health care professions.

THE NURSE AS PART OF THE CHEMICAL DEPENDENCY TREATMENT TEAM

The treatment of chemical dependency is usually conducted by a multidisciplinary or an interdisciplinary team, which includes nurses. Nurses choose chemical dependency treatment work for a variety of reasons. Some are drawn by virtue of their own recovery or the recovery of someone they love. Others work with chemically dependent patients to achieve the same satisfaction that they derive from working with patients with other illnesses. Most lack formal preparation, regardless of their educational background. Additionally, there is wide variation in nurses' roles among treatment programs. Some providers limit nurses to managing patients during withdrawal, monitoring physical problems, medication side effects, and vital signs, and administering occasional medications. Other programs employ nurses as primary therapists. Nurses also function as middle- and upper-level managers in many treatment programs.

Nurses who are limited to caring for patients in the detoxification phase are usually frustrated. Most nurses want to work with patients and their families during all aspects of recovery. Because of the limitation of these programs, it is not unusual for nurses to leave the structure of nursing for the position of counselor. They can retain their license to practice nursing, but their affiliation moves to the chemical dependency field.

Nurses who are educated and experienced in the treatment of chemical dependency have special skills that most of the treatment team does not possess, including an understanding of the physiological processes during detoxification and through recovery. Many patients and their families will talk with nurses when they will not talk with other treatment team members about a variety of problems, fears, and concerns. Nurses have extensive experience in communicating with other professionals about patient care.

As education about chemical dependency improves, so must the preparation of nurses. Other professionals in chemical dependency also must learn more about the value nurses can add to the multidisciplinary team, to appropriately utilize the nurse's training and ability. There should be an opportunity for professional challenge and satisfaction within a nursing role.

RECOMMENDED IMPROVEMENTS IN ASSISTANCE TO CHEMICALLY DEPENDENT NURSES

Most nurses still do not know about chemical dependency services, and those who do may receive inadequate or mistimed assistance. A more comprehensive approach must be developed to identify nurses in the early stages of their disease, intervene appropriately, and, most importantly, follow them through the long and difficult reentry process.

Several methods of providing more comprehensive and consistent assistance are recommended. Peer assistance programs provided by state nurses' associations and/or state boards of nursing are most likely to be staffed by paid professionals. These professionals should be truly knowledgeable about the field of chemical dependency. A paid staff will be more likely to make a long-term commitment to the program than a volunteer staff. Also, a professional staff may have more control over the preparation, credentials, and training of those who will be assisting vulnerable people. These professional standards are difficult to maintain with volunteers, no matter how well intentioned they are. A professional staff has the power to influence creatively a nurse's career, and therefore the lines of authority, responsibility, and accountability must be clearly delineated. The staff must have the resources to to an adequate job.

We credit the trailblazing volunteers who have given unselfishly of their time to educate their colleagues and assist fellow nurses. Their initial efforts are responsible for the assistance programs in existence today. We must now formalize and permanently establish these programs with the continued assistance and participation of those pioneers. Thus we can continue to benefit from their talent, energy, and dedication.

In addition to formal assistance programs, the link between institutional employee assistance programs and nursing assistance groups should be strengthened. Nurses have been reluctant to use EAPs, fearing that confidentiality would not be maintained and that they would lose jobs or nursing licenses. EAP personnel should receive education about the legal issues involved in treating and referring nurses and other licensed professionals (see Chapter 6). Networking among EAP personnel, nursing administrators, and nursing assistance programs could benefit all parties by promoting an understanding of parallel functions, legal considerations, and potential cooperative working arrangements.

Finally, state boards of nursing and assistance programs should develop stronger working relationships. Florida, Texas, California, and New Mexico have mandated peer assistance programs. With these programs, if the nurse is successful with recovery, disciplinary action is not undertaken. Although not required by state law, other states have established agreements between the state board of nursing and the state nurse's association to refer chemically dependent nurses to the assistance program before taking further action. This combination of regulation and assistance can provide the necessary structure while maintaining support.

POLICY DEVELOPMENT

The American Nursing Association (ANA) continues to address policies related to nurses whose professional functioning is impaired by chemical dependency. A special committee, including representation from the National Nurses' Society on Addictions (NNSA) and the Drug and Alcohol Nursing Association (DANA), is directing these activities. The ANA Council on Psychiatric and Mental Health Nursing established a Task Force on Substance Abuse Nursing Practice. The work of the task force has been published as "The Case of Clients with Addictions: Dimensions of Nursing Practice" (ANA: Kansas City, MO, 1987). A separate task force representing both groups will soon publish standards of care. Furthermore, the NNSA has a subcommittee on nurses' addictions. All of these national nursing organizations are concerned about chemical dependency and are moving to address the problem by developing policy recommendations. These efforts must continue and they must be used to influence legislation as well as the policy and procedures adopted by institutions. The groundwork for implementation of the recommended policies is being laid by these organizational efforts. Nursing organizations' efforts in addressing the problem are listed in Appendix C.

   Assistance to nurses has only just begun. The profession is beginning to establish assistance and research programs and is increasing its efforts to initiate policy and legislation. Efforts must continue in all these areas, and educational programs must be developed so that every nurse is presented with basic information about the disease and guidelines for action should personal chemical dependency problems develop. Nurses' lives, those of their colleagues, and their professional futures depend on it. The health and safety of our patients mandate it.

ADDENDUM

FOR THE CHEMICALLY DEPENDENT NURSE

IF YOU THINK OR KNOW YOU HAVE A PROBLEM

The first step in solving a problem is to acknowledge it exists! The universal pattern in chemical dependency is to rationalize, delay, and deny rather than to overdiagnose and jump to conclusions. Do not ignore your suspicions, whether they concern yourself or someone else. It is easier and more comfortable to do nothing, particularly if the alternative is a long, hard look in the mirror. Many of us are reluctant to upset other people by bringing up the subject.

There are many self-tests to identify alcoholism. The two most widely accepted are the CAGE and MAST tests. The former consists of only four questions; the latter has both a long and a short version. (These tests may be found in Appendix J.) There are also tests available to help assess whether you are having problems due to a family member's addiction. You may be "co-dependent," preventing or interfering with someone's recovery rather than helping it progress.

If the results of the tests indicate that there is a problem, or if doubt remains, it is time for action. To do nothing or to try to handle a potential chemical dependency problem on one's own is rarely advisable. If the problem involves a lover or a family member, do not attempt home remedies. You did not cause the problem and you cannot cure it alone. You *are* responsible for finding treatment. Chemical dependents are adept at convincing themselves that someone or something else is to blame for their difficulties and at making others feel responsible. They also use past tragedies and life situations as excuses for their present problems. With those rationalizations, it is easy to believe it impossible or unreasonable to expect the drinking or other drug use to stop. All concerned become paralyzed and nothing changes.

When the problem is your own, you need only review your own experience to know that good resolutions, a bigger dose of willpower and sincere attempts to change are not enough to overcome the situation. You want to believe that you are still in control and can manage on your own. It is true that most alcoholics are able to control their drinking most of the time, just as cocaine addicts can sometimes stop with one line. The perception that one cannot always predict in advance how much one is going to drink or use or, if one is not currently drinking or using, when one will start again is the key to recognizing loss of control. It is not a question of keeping promises to others. What's lost is the ability to keep those secret promises made to oneself. If every drinking occasion resulted in humiliation, guilt, or disaster, denial would shatter easily. While things go well, you can maintain the delusion that all will work out for you without major changes.

Since "do it yourself" solutions usually fail, what else is possible? Obvious resources include the mutual help groups like Alcoholics Anonymous (AA), Narcotics Anonymous (NA), and Al-Anon. If you live anywhere in the United States or Canada, you will probably have a choice of AA groups; in Great Britain there are fewer groups. Almost everyone initially feels self-conscious about approaching these groups and may be concerned about gossip. If you live in a very small town, you may want to attend introductory meetings out of town. If you are worried and wary, be aware that AA groups have both "open" meetings and "closed" meetings; the former open to anyone who wants to visit and learn about AA (including health care professionals concerned about patients and colleagues) and the latter limited to those who know or believe they are alcoholic.

You will not be asked to sign anything and you need not give your last name. Other participants will understand your feelings better than anyone; they have been in your place. All participants are expected to keep confidential anything they learn of a personal nature, including the names of the participants. AA prefers to remain self-supporting, so the group prefers that visitors do not contribute when the basket is passed to collect for group expenses.

If you do not want to join AA, there are a variety of local councils on alcoholism, many of them affiliated with the National Council on Alcoholism (1-800-NCA-CALL). A few of these groups provide counseling, however, most help people find other resources. The local councils usually are good sources of information about available outpatient counseling as well as hospitals and treatment centers for alcohol and other drug abuse.

Most telephone books list a surprising array of treatment possibilities under alcoholism in the Yellow Pages. Ask about fees, insurance, whether the facility is approved by the Joint Commission for Accreditation of Hospitals. Does the facility urge you to admit yourself for residential care or do they attempt to learn whether or not you need and can profit from what they offer? It is very important to choose a place that specializes in or places heavy emphasis on alcoholism and other addictions rather than a more generic mental health setting where this expertise is usually lacking. It is always tempting to look for the "why" of addiction rather than the "how" of recovery. If you and your therapist are committed to that wild goose chase of "why," you can continue drinking or taking drugs while hoping that insight or learning new coping skills will miraculously effect a cure.[1]

In general, it makes sense to try simple measures first. If AA alone does not solve the problem, move on rapidly to a discussion with a knowledgeable professional. A professional's academic credentials are not as important as skill and experience in treating chemical dependency. The best person may be a nurse, a social worker, a psychiatrist, a certified alcohol or drug counselor or someone from yet another discipline. If outpatient care does not help or if your counselor feels strongly that residential care is needed, accept that judgment and enter a residential program. In general, alcoholics and other addicts try to expend minimal effort and time to recover from their illness and they continue to underestimate the lethal nature of their disease. Alcoholism or other drug addiction *is* a legitimate illness that needs expert care

---

[1]Understanding and new skills are better learned *after* one's head is clear of chemicals; problems can then be evaluated without the confounding effects of drugs.

now, not when all your other obligations and concerns have been settled. If you had an acute myocardial infarction you would not refuse to enter a coronary care unit because you first needed to prepare the children for camp. Do not delay, no matter what plausible excuses you can find.

Do you need to go to a special facility for nurses or to a nurses' support or treatment group in addition to AA? This issue has been hotly debated. Some feel that only another nurse can understand; others have said that the last one they want to share this problem with is another nurse. Many nurses have recovered in a variety of settings. The common denominators emerge as an honest acknowledgement of the addiction, acceptance of the need for abstinence from alcohol and all other mood-altering drugs, and ongoing involvement with a long-term support system after initial treatment.

Although concrete documentation is incomplete, the prognosis for recovery is good and there is reason for optimism. Just do not delay and do not deny. If simple measures are not effective and you continue to drink or use other drugs, promptly arrange for more intensive care. Conventional wisdom holds that "If it's working, don't fix it!" but we must add, "If it's not working, face it and fix it!"

IF YOU ARE IN TREATMENT

Perhaps you are reading this while still in treatment and imagining what it will be like to go home and "face the music." If you have kept your treatment secret, you may need to decide what, if anything, to reveal to others and where to get follow-up care. Or you may be in the opposite situation; you may have been led out of a hospital in hand-cuffs. Either way, there will be decisions to make and dilemmas to solve.

If there are legal problems to confront concerning child custody, divorce, malpractice, or your license, you will need professional advice. Decisions about your future may be delayed and may often seem unfair. Remember how little you knew about chemical dependency before you entered treatment and realize that many of your colleagues and those in a position to decide your future may not have much knowledge about the subject either. Some people will be wise, aware, and compassionate and others will have little understanding of your plight. You may need to draw on your reserves of patience when your impulse is to rush back into harness and prove to everyone that all is well and that you can be the best nurse in the region. Do not try to be perfect overnight. It is a significant accomplishment to be drug-free and sober and, above all, predictable and reliable.

If you face both criminal charges and board hearings, arrange to confront the criminal charges first. Minimize your culpability; let others prove your guilt. In a board hearing, however, candor may work to your advantage. If you level with the board members, they may be more supportive. Unfortunately, if they do rule against you, the law may make your record publically available and hence accessible by the courts. If you handle the courts first and the board second, you can be more open and honest with the board. Remember that the board's primary responsibility is to protect the public from unsafe practitioners.

If there is a local nurses' support group, use it to test the local climate before you decide what and to whom to confide. Do not make assumptions; you may discover that your news is not news to others. You may be accepted back into the profession quite fairly and fully. You may also find yourself under suspicion. Remember that it is not humanly possible to be sober for two years after two weeks of treatment. It will take time to demonstrate that you can be trusted, that you are not just behaving well while under observation.

Treatment does not end when you leave a hospital or residential treatment center. Do not leave your addiction only partially treated, whether you think you can handle it yourself or not. If you have been told to go to AA or NA, go there. Get a sponsor. Go regularly and get involved with the group; do not just sit in the back row. Give these meetings the same importance as other major commitments like working and caring for family. If you relapse, all of the other aspects of your life will deteriorate anyway. If you are assigned to outpatient treatment, honor that commitment as well.

Do not cut corners and do not try to make up for past sins by shortchanging yourself. It will be tempting to commit to a double shift when you are expected at a group session or an AA meeting, particularly when you feel vulnerable. Your primary responsibility is to invest the necessary time and effort in your recovery.

Hundreds of nurses have recovered successfully in spite of personal horror stories. The long-term prognosis is good; the most important step toward recovery is not to pick up the first glass, syringe, or pill. Take your time and let others take theirs.

WORKING IN THE FIELD

During your treatment, you may consider making a career change to work full time with alcoholics and other addicts. Patients are often eager to work as alcoholism counselors almost from the moment they leave treatment. During the honeymoon period, it may seem like a grand idea to share one's experience and new understanding with patients and colleagues either as therapist or even as teacher of other nurses. It may indeed be a good idea, but resist such impulses until you have solidly resolved your own problem and achieved a comfortable reentry to the "outside world." Working with alcoholics and other addicts places you in a setting where there is a common culture and understanding; the battle of survival in nursing should not be avoided. If you avoid the reentry problem, you have not really finished working through your own problems.

Chemical dependency counselors are generally not hired with less than two to three years of sobriety. Begin by learning about your disease and about the workings of AA and NA. Work with others in your group as soon as the group feels you are ready, but delay plunging into this work full-time. Think about alcoholism and addiction, the roles of being nurse and being a patient and about your ability to delay gratification. Then make your plans, short-term and long-term. We wish you the best of luck.

Selected References

Readings

Ackerman, R. (1983). *Children of alcoholics.* Holmes Beach, FL: Learning Publications Press.

Alcoholics Anonymous. (1976). New York: Alcoholics Anonymous World Services, Inc.

American Nurses' Association. (1984). *Addiction and psychological dysfunction in nursing: The profession's response to the problem.* Kansas City, MO: ANA.

Beckman, L.J. (1975). Women alcoholics: A review of social and psychological studies. *Journal of Studies on Alcohol,* 36(7), 797–824.

Beckman, L.J. (1978). Self-esteem of women alcoholics. *Journal of Studies on Alcohol,* 39(3), 491–498.

Bennett, G., Vourakis, C., & Woolf, D. (1983). *Substance abuse: Pharmacologic, developmental, and clinical perspectives.* New York: John Wiley & Sons.

Berry, C.A. (1981). *Good health for employees and reduced health care for industry.* Washington, DC: Health Insurance Association of America.

Bissell, L., & Haberman, P.W. (1984). *Alcoholism in the professions.* New York: Oxford University Press.

Bissell, L., & Jones, R.W. (1981). The alcoholic nurse. *Nursing Outlook,* 29(2), 96–100.

Bissell, L. & Royce, J.E. (1987) *Ethics for Addiction Professionals.* Center City, MN: Hazelden Foundation.

Bissell, L., & Skorina, J. (1987, June 5). 100 alcoholic women in medicine. *JAMA,* 257(21), 2939–2944.

Black, C. (1981). *It will never happen to me.* Denver: M.A.C.

Black, C. (1985). *Repeat after me.* Denver: M.A.C.

Blume, S. (1986, June 17). *Women and alcohol.* National Conference on Women's Health.

Brennan, L. (1983). *The recovering alcoholically impaired nurse: A descriptive study.* Unpublished master's thesis, Rutgers University, New Brunswick, NJ.

Brown, S. (1985). *Treating the alcoholic: A developmental model of recovery.* New York: John Wiley & Sons.

Cermak, T. (1986, April). Diagnostic criteria for co-dependency. *Digest of Addiction Theory and Application,* 5(3), 5–13.

Collins, S. (1984). *EAP: Annual report of cost savings, 1983–1984.* Unpublished report, The Jewish Hospital of St. Louis.

Corrigan, E.M. (1980). *Alcoholic women in treatment.* New York: Oxford University Press.

Dackis, C.A., Gold, M.S., Pottash, A.L.C., & Sweeney, D.R. (1986). Evaluating depression in alcoholics. *Psychiatric Research,* 17(2), 105–109.

DaDalt, R.A. (1986, July). Changing patterns of drug diversion. *The American Journal of Nursing,* 86(7), 792–794.

Dean, P., & Edwards, T. (1986). *Adult children of alcoholics.* The First National Conference for Research and Study on Substance Abuse in Nursing, Atlanta, GA.

DeSoto, C.B., O'Donnell, W.E., Alfred, L.J., & Lopes, C.E. (1985). Symptomatology in alcoholics at various stages of abstinence. *Alcoholism: Clinical and Experimental Research,* 9(6), 505–512.

Edens, K., Muldoon, J. Sternou, R., & Murck, M. (1987). *How to use intervention in your profession.* Minneapolis: Johnson Institute.

Ellis, G.M., Jr., Mann, M.A., Judson, B.A., Schramm, N.,T., & Tashcian, A. (1985). Excretion patterns of cannabinoid metabolites after last use in a group of chronic users. *Clinical Pharmacologic Therapeutics,* 38(5), 572–578.

Estes, N.J. & Heineman, M.E. (1986). *Alcoholism: Development, consequence and interventions* (3rd ed.). St. Louis: C.V. Mosby.

Finnegan, D.G. (1987). *Dual identities: counseling chemically dependent gay men and lesbians.* Center City, MN: Hazelden.

Ford, B., & Chase, C. (1987). *Betty, a glad awakening.* Garden City, NY: Doubleday.

Gitlow, S.E., & Peyser, H.S. (Eds.). (1980). *Alcoholism, a practical treatment guide.* New York: Grune and Stratton.

Glaser, F.B., & Ogborne, A.C. (1982). Does AA really work? *British Journal of Addictions, 77*(2), 123–129.

Glatt, M.M. (1968, February 10). Alcoholism and drug dependence in doctors and nurses. *British Medical Journal, 1*(5588), 380–381.

Glatt, M.M. (1976). Alcoholism an occupational hazard for doctors. *Journal of Alcoholism, 11*, 85–91.

Goodwin, D.W. (1981). Alcoholism and heredity. *Journal of the National Association of Private Psychiatric Hospitals, 12*, 94–96.

Graves, J. (1982, April). Orem's self-care concept of nursing practice: Use with recovering alcoholics and co-alcoholics. *The Proceedings of the 1982 Annual Conference of the National Nurses Society on Alcoholism.* Washington, DC.

Haack, M.R. & Hughes, T.L. (Eds.). (1988). *Impairment in nursing: Clinical perspectives and program development.* New York: Springer.

Haack, M.R. & Harford, T.C. (1984). Drinking patterns among student nurses. *International Journal of the Addictions, 19*(5), 577–583.

Hasin, D., Endicott, J., & Lewis, C. (1985). Alcohol and drug abuse in patients with affective syndromes. *Comprehensive Psychiatry, 26*(3), 283–295.

Hesselbrock, M.N., Meyer, R.E., & Keener, J.J. (1985). Psychopathology in hospitalized alcoholics. *Archives of General Psychiatry, 42*(11), 1050–1055.

Hoffman, F.M. (1985). Cost per RN hired. *Journal of Nursing Administration, 15*(2), 27–29.

Holder, H.D., Blose, J.O., & Gasiorowski, M.J. (1985). *Alcoholism treatment impact on total health care utilization and costs: A four-year longitudinal analysis of the federal employees' health benefit program with Aetna Life Insurance Company* (NTIS No. PB-86-18757). Chapel Hill, NC.

Hutchinson, S. (1986). Chemically dependent nurses: The trajectory toward self-annihilation. *Nursing Research, 35*(4), 196–201.

Jaffe, S. (1982, April). Help for the helper: Firsthand views of recovery. *American Journal of Nursing, 82*(4), 578–579.

Jefferson, L., & Ensor, B. (1982, April). Confronting a chemically-impaired colleague. *American Journal of Nursing, 82*(4), 574-576.

Jellinek, E.M. (1960). *The disease concept of alcoholism.* New Haven, CT: College and University Press.

Johnson, V. (1986). *Intervention: How to help someone who doesn't want help.* Minneapolis: Johnson Institute.

Johnson, V.E. (1973). *I'll quit tomorrow.* New York: Harper & Row.

Kelley, R.D. (1985). Rx: Swifter help for chemically dependent nurses. *American Journal of Nursing,* 85(6), 640–641.

Kelly, L.S. (1986). Shadows on the image. (Editorial). *Nursing Outlook,* 34(5), 219.

Kilburg, R.R., Nathan, P.E., & Thoreson, R.N. (1986). *Professionals in distress: Issues, syndromes, and solutions in psychology.* Washington, DC: American Psychological Association.

King, Barbara. (1986, Fall). Decision making in the intervention process. *Alcoholism Treatment Quarterly,* 3(3), 5–22.

Kline, R.B., & Snyder, D.K. (1985). Replicated MMPI subtypes for alcoholic men and women: Relationship to self-reported drinking behaviors. *Journal of Consulting and Clinical Psychology,* 53(1), 70–79.

Kornblum, A. (1987, January 23/30). Working an uneasy truce. *American Medical News,* pp. 17, 18, 20.

Kurtz, E. (1982). Why AA works: The intellectual significance of AA. *Journal of Studies on Alcohol,* 43(1), 38–80.

Levine, D.G., Preston, P.A., & Lipscomb, S.G. (1974). A historical approach to understanding drug abuse among nurses. *American Journal of Psychiatry,* 131(9), 1036–1037.

Martin, E. (1987). *Breaking the Cycle.* New York: Harper & Row.

Maxwell, M.A. (1962). Alcoholics Anonymous: An interpretation. In D.J. Pittman and C.R. Snyder (Eds.), *Society, culture, and drinking patterns* (pp. 577–585). New York: John Wiley & Sons.

Maxwell, M.A. (1984). *The AA experience.* New York: McGraw-Hill.

McAuliffe, W.E., Rohman, M., Santangelo, S.L., Feldman, B., Magnuson, E., Sobol, A., & Weissman, J. (1986). Psychoactive drug use among practicing physicians and medical students. *New England Journal of Medicine,* 315(13), 805–810.

McAuliffe, W.E., Santangelo, S.L., Gingras, J., Rohman, M., Sobol, A., & Magnuson, E. (1987). Use and abuse of controlled substances by pharmacists and pharmacy students. *American Journal of Hospital Pharmacy,* 44(2), 311–317.

McCaun, J. (1986). Hospital security consultant outlines methods employees use for diverting narcotic drugs. *Oncology Times,* 9(2), 28–30.

McGuire, F.B. (1987). Philosophy from Flo. *Newsletter of the Missouri State Board of Nursing,* 28(1), 2–3.

Morse, R.M., Martin, M.A., Swenson, W.M., & Niven, R.G. (1984, February 10). Prognosis of physicians treated for alcoholism and drug dependence. *Journal of the American Medical Association*, 251(6), 743–746.

Murray, P.M. (1976, October 2). Alcoholism among male doctors in Scotland. *Lancet*, 7988(2), 729–731.

Naegle, M.A. (1987). Disclosure or silence on impaired practice? (Letter to the editor). *Nursing Outlook*, 35(1), 9.

National Council of State Boards of Nursing. (1980–1981). *Preliminary sample of board actions.* Unpublished data.

Nichols, M. (1985). Theoretical concerns in the clinical treatment of substance-abusing women: A feminist analysis. *Alcoholism Treatment Quarterly*, 2(1), 79–90. (Special issue: Psychosocial issues in the treatment of alcoholism)

O'Briant, R., & Lennard, H. (1973). *Recovery from alcoholism.* Springfield, IL: Charles C. Thomas.

Orem, D.E. (1985). *Nursing: Concepts of practice.* New York: McGraw-Hill.

Pendery, M.L., Maltzman, I.M., & West, L.J. (1982). Controlled drinking by alcoholics? New findings and a reevaluation of a major affirmative study. *Science*, 217(4555), 169–175.

Penny, J.T. (1986). Spotlight on support for impaired nurses. *American Journal of Nursing*, 86(3), 689–691.

Perrin, T. (1983, July-August). (Editorial). *COA Review*, p. 2.

Pokorney, A.D., & Solomon, J. (1983). Follow-up survey of drug abuse and alcoholism teaching in medical schools. *Journal of Medical Education*, 58, 316–321.

Poplar, J.F. (1969). Characteristics of nurse addicts. *American Journal of Nursing*, 69, 117–119.

Reed, M. (1986). Descriptive study of chemically dependent nurses. In J. Brooking (Ed.), *Psychiatric nursing research* (pp. 157–173). New York: John Wiley & Sons.

Royce, J. (1981). *Alcohol problems and alcoholism.* New York: Free Press.

Scanlon, W.F. (1986). *Alcoholism and drug abuse in the workplace: Employee assistance programs.* New York: Praeger Publishers.

Schaef, A.W. (1986). *Misunderstood, mistreated.* Minneapolis: Winston Press.

Sullivan, E.J. (1986, July-August). Cost savings of retaining chemically dependent nurses. *Nursing Economics*, 4(4), 179–182, 200.

Sullivan, E.J. (1987a). A descriptive study of nurses recovering from chemical dependency. *Archives of Psychiatric Nursing*, 1(3), 194–200.

Sullivan, E.J. (1987b). Comparison of chemically dependent and non-dependent nurses on familial, personal, and professional characteristics. *Journal of Studies on Alcohol,* 48(6), 563–568.

Taylor, R.A., Weisman, A.P., & Gest, T. (1986, July 28). America on drugs. *U.S. News & World Report,* pp. 48–54.

Thyer, B. (1986). Alcohol abuse among clinically anxious patients. *Behavior Research and Therapy,* 24(3), 357–359.

U.S. Department of Health and Human Services, National Institute on Alcohol Abuse and Alcoholism. (1983, December). *Fifth special report to the U.S. Congress on alcohol and health.* Washington, DC: Government Printing Office.

Wegscheider, S. (1983, November/December). Co-dependency: The therapeutic void. *Focus on the Family and Chemical Dependency,* 6(6).

Wood, P.J. (1985). Evidence of alcoholism among professional nurses: What colleagues report (Doctoral dissertation, University of Michigan). *Dissertation Abstracts International,* 46(7), 378.

AUDIO-VISUALS

Grandview Hospital and Medical Center (Producer), & Johnson, E. (Director). (1986). *Chemical Dependency and nurses: The deadly secret* (Videocassette). Dayton, OH: Grandview Hospital and Medical Center Media Productions.

Johnson Institute (Producer). (1976). *I'll quit tomorrow* (Videocassette). Minneapolis: Johnson Institute.

Johnson Institute (Producer). (1979). *The enablers* (Videocassette). Minneapolis: Johnson Institute.

Johnson Institute (Producer). (1979). *The intervention* (Videocassette). Minneapolis: Johnson Institute.

Public Relations Department of Ridgeview Institute (Producer), & Verdery, V.L., & O'Sullivan, P. (Directors). (1984). *Intervention: Rescue from destruction* (Videocassette). Smyrna, GA: Ridgeview Institute.

Public Relations Department of Ridgeview Institute (Producer), & Verdery, V.L., & O'Sullivan, P. (Directors). (1986). *Addiction, R.N.* (Videocassette). Smyrna, GA: Ridgeview Institute.

APPENDIX A

Model Curriculum Outline On Chemical Dependency Among Nurses

I. Information on chemical dependency
   A. Incidence
      1. Demographic differences
      2. Special populations
   B. Definition of chemical dependency
      1. Quantity, frequency and pattern of use
      2. Life problems definition
      3. Criteria for diagnosis of chemical dependency
   C. Etiology
      1. Genetic predisposition
      2. Family influences
      3. Social factors
   D. Disease progression
      1. Physical deterioration
      2. Emotional and social effects
   E. Assessment of chemical dependency
      1. Physical and psychological criteria
         a. increasing use and tolerance
         b. physiological damage
         c. life problems
         d. withdrawal

F. Intervention
   1. Medical treatment
   2. Nursing diagnosis
   3. Behavioral approach
   4. Types of treatment
      a. inpatient
      b. outpatient
      c. aftercare
      d. halfway house
      e. supplemental counseling
   5. Treating other psychiatric/psychological problems
   along with chemical dependency

G. Attitudes toward chemical dependency
   1. Societal
   2. Health professionals
   3. Stigma for women, nurses, narcotics' users, men in
   nursing

H. Denial
   1. In addicted person
   2. In colleagues/families/friends
   3. In the profession

II. Nurses with chemical dependency

A. Incidence among nurses
   1. State board reports
   2. Estimates

B. Special characteristics of nurses
   1. Common use of pharmaceuticals
   2. Lack of education regarding chemical dependency
   3. Stress of work setting
   4. Stigma

C. Identification
   1. Types of drugs used
      a. narcotics
      b. alcohol
      c. tranquilizers and sedatives
      d. stimulants
      e. hallucinogens
   2. Type and place of use
      a. on-the-job use
      b. recreational use
      c. therapeutic use
   3. Signs and symptoms
   4. Job performance changes

    D. Intervention
        1. Job setting intervention
            a. peer/colleagues
            b. supervisor/employer
        2. Steps in intervention
            a. caring attitude
            b. be prepared
            c. have referral sources available
            d. know consequences and be prepared to follow through

    E. Treatment
        1. Selection of facility
            a. sensitivity to nurses' problems
            b. costs and insurance coverage
            c. philosophy
        2. Goals of treatment
            a. abstinence from all mood-altering chemicals
            b. reentry to nursing

    F. Reentry issues
        1. Contingency contracts
            a. monitoring
            b. random urine screens
        2. Individualized assignments
            a. controlled substances' administration
            b. rotating shifts
            c. what to tell/not tell the staff

III. Legal and ethical issues

    A. Nurses' rights vs. patient/public responsibility

    B. Institutional liability
        1. Patient injury
        2. Wrongful termination
        3. Discrimination based on handicap

    C. Nurse Practice Act
        1. Violations
        2. Reporting
        3. Licensure sanctions

    D. Criminal justice system

IV. Future needs
   A. Institutional/agency policies for intervention, treatment and reentry
   B. Education
      1. Schools of nursing
      2. Inservice education
      3. Continuing education
   C. Legislation to provide treatment before discipline
   D. Research
      1. To know what assists nurses with recovery
      2. Determine risk factors for prevention planning
      3. Evaluate assistance program

APPENDIX B

RESOLUTIONS RELATED TO CHEMICAL DEPENDENCY AMONG NURSES

AMERICAN NURSES' ASSOCIATION

Resolution 5: Action on Alcohol and Drug Misuse and Psychological Dysfunctions among Nurses

Adopted June 29, 1982 by ANA House of Delegates

WHEREAS, There are people in the United States among whom are registered nurses whose functioning is impaired because of misuse of alcohol and other drugs or because of emotional and psychological dysfunction; and

WHEREAS, The membership of the American Nurses' Association recognizes its professional responsibility to colleagues and to those they serve; and

WHEREAS, Misuse of alcohol and other drugs and emotional and psychological dysfunction can impair the individual's ability to meet the requirements of the Code for Nurses; and

WHEREAS, Timely and effective intervention can contribute to the restoration to health of the nurse, the maintenance of standards for nursing practice, adherence to the Code for Nurses, and the safety of the public; therefore, be it

RESOLVED, That ANA, in collaboration with other health care organizations and interested groups, develop guidelines for establishing programs of assistance and intervention for those nurses whose functioning is impaired because of misuse of alcohol and other drugs or because of emotional and psychological dysfunction; and be it

RESOLVED, That ANA encourage nursing administrators and other employers of nurses to offer appropriate treatment antecedent to disciplinary action in the same manner as with other health problems and to maintain options for continuing or subsequent employment; and be it

RESOLVED, That ANA establish mechanisms for continuing collection and dissemination of information that includes statistical data, status of program implementation, significant educational and research activities, and legal and ethical issues as related to the impaired nurse.

Source: American Nurses' Association. *Summary of Proceedings.* Kansas City, MO.: American Nurses' Association, 1983. Used with permission.

NATIONAL LEAGUE FOR NURSING

Resolution 4: For Developing Programs for Nurses Who Are Impaired by Substance Abuse

Adopted June 3, 1983 by the NLN Membership at the 16th Biennial Convention

WHEREAS, Chemical (alcohol and drug) dependency is a complicated disease with physical and psychosocial components and with unfavorable economic consequences for the individual and society; and

WHEREAS, Nurses along with other health professionals, are exposed to many risks of developing the disease; and

WHEREAS, Chemical dependency can impair professional competence for maintaining standards of care and protecting the public; and

WHEREAS, A profession must be accountable for monitoring and regulating its own membership; and

WHEREAS, The membership of the NLN recognizes its professional obligations to colleagues and those they serve; therefore, be it

RESOLVED, That NLN encourage schools of nursing and health care institutions to provide educational programs on chemical dependence among health professionals, and be it further

RESOLVED, That NLN provide information to its membership through its official publication regarding established programs and resources to assist substance abusers.

APPENDIX C

NATIONAL NURSING ORGANIZATIONS' ACTIVITIES RELATED TO CHEMICAL DEPENDENCY

ORGANIZATION AND ACTIVITIES

National Association of School Nurses (NASN)

1. No program in place re: chemical dependency.

2. Provided a speaker on "The Impaired Nurse" at 1987 annual conference in Chicago.

National Federation of Licensed Practical Nurses, Inc. (NFLPN)

1. Works with other health care associations and interested parties to encourage the establishment of programs of assistance for LP/VN's.

2. Encourages its member states to establish assistance programs that will aid LPN's to obtain treatment while maintaining a position in leave status so insurance and other reimbursements will assist with the costs.

3. Offers continuing education at national conventions that focus on high-risk factors for impairments among LPN's.

4. NFLPN Practice Standards include statements that address responsibility for professional conduct.

American Association of Occupational Health Nurses (AAOHN)

1. Developed a position statement regarding impaired nursing practice.

2. Provided professional development programs on the subject.

National Association for Practical Nurse Education and Service (NAPNES)

Published an article on this subject in December 87 issue of *The Journal of Practical Nursing.*

Association of Rehabilitation Nurses (ARN)

Developed a position statement on the impaired nurse.

American Association of Critical Care Nurses (AACN)

1. Publishes articles periodically directed toward chemically dependent nurses and related problems.

2. Offered a forum at the 1987 National Teaching Institute entitled, "The Manager's Dilemma; Employee Substance Abuse."

American Hospital Association (AHA)

1. AHA Media Center produced teleconference 1/87 entitled, "Drug Testing in Hospitals: Access or Liability?"

2. AHA Public Relations department is producing a substance abuse kit for use in public and member communication.

3. AHA cosponsored a conference program titled, "Management of the Impaired Health Professional: Educating Ourselves and Educating Others," October, 1987.

Nurses' Association, American College of Obstetricians and Gynecologists (NAACOG)

1. Feature article in newsletter, "Nurses' Special Chemical Dependency Problems," November, 1985.

2. No formal program.

National Student Nurses' Association (NSNA)

1. Provided education programs on chemical dependency at conventions.

2. Passed resolutions by 1983 House of Delegates entitled, "Support of Drug and Alcohol Impaired Nurse Programs" and "Nursing Students' Need for Education on Alcoholism."

National Nurses Society on Addictions (NNSA)

1. Established and continues to support a national network of nurses available to contact nurses who are experiencing problems with alcohol/drugs or are new in recovery.

2. Published statement on Model Diversion Legislation for Chemically Impaired Nurses.

3. Developed a position paper on "The Impaired Nurses."

4. Maintains up-to-date list of activities in each state in regard to impaired nurse programs.

5. Maintains representation on the American Nurses Association Impaired Nurse Committee.

6. Sponsors educational programs on the impaired nurse issues.

National Association of Pediatric Nurse Associates & Practitioners

Nothing offered at this time.

American Organization of Nurse Executives (AONE)

Nothing offered.

American Society of Post Anesthesia Nurses (ASPAN)

1. Each year at the national conference (usually April), a lecture session addressing the issue is presented.

2. In 4/87 Marshall Wilkerson presented lecture at L.A. conference "Substance Abuse in the Profession."

American Association of Nurse Anesthetists (AANA)

1. Policy statement

2. Manual on chemical dependency

3. CD coordinators for each state (state level)

4. AANA appointed Peer Assistance advisor (national level)

5. CD hotline

The Association of Operating Room Nurses (AORN)

>   No services provided.

Emergency Nurses Association (ENA)

>   No services provided.

National Association of Orthopedic Nurses (NAON)

>   No formal programs at this time.

National Nursing Organizations' Position Statements on Addictions

National Nurses' Society on Addictions Position Paper: The Impaired Nurse

The National Nurses' Society on Addictions—(NNSA), as a professional organization of nurses with specialized interest and expertise in the field of chemical dependency, has adopted the following statement in regard to the nurse whose professional performance has become impaired due to the use of mind-altering chemicals.

This position paper grew out of a concern by the members of NNSA that the profession is losing nurses through the revocation of licensure and that, furthermore, before the chemical dependency progresses to the point of disciplinary action, the well-being of their patients is being jeopardized. At the NNSA Forum in April, 1982, the membership discussed the issues involved with the stated purpose of arriving at an official position in regard to this most serious problem.

While recognizing that nurses can become impaired due to physical or mental illness as well as chemical dependency, NNSA believes that chemical dependency is by far the greater problem. By fashioning a mechanism for identifying and intervening in cases of chemical dependency, other problems of impairment can be handled as well.

In its position statement, "Role of the Nurse in Alcoholism," ratified in 1979, NNSA affirmed its belief that alcoholism is a primary disease. Alcoholism is but one manifestation of the disease process of addiction to a chemical; that of addiction to alcohol. The scope of this paper includes addiction (or chemical dependency as it is frequently termed) to any mind-altering drug; both physiological and psychological dependency. The definition of chemical dependency is the continued use of any mind-altering drug (or combination of drugs) to the extent that such use interferes with function in important areas of a person's life.

Since chemical dependency is a disease process, the nurse is no more immune from falling victim to it than he or she would be from any other disease. Although exact figures on the extent of drug dependency among nurses are not known, one widely accepted figure for alcoholic nurses places the number at 40,000 out of 1.6 million licensed nurses. The National Council of State Boards of Nursing compiled data from its member state boards and determined that during the period from September, 1980 to August, 1981, 67% or 649 disciplinary actions were for substance abuse. Since the profession of nursing is highly reluctant to identify problems with chemical dependency until the process is well advanced, this number could be greatly enlarged if nurses who quit or are terminated before their use of alcohol and/or drugs becomes blatant were counted. The number of 649 is but the tip of the iceberg.

NNSA affirms its belief that the nursing profession bears a threefold responsibility in regard to this problem. First of all, nursing is responsible for assuring that no patient be placed in jeopardy due to the unrecognized and untreated illness of a nurse. Secondly, there is a responsibility to maintain standards of integrity and practice within the profession. Nursing must engage in self-regulation as a part of ethical practice. And thirdly, there is a responsibility to the welfare of the individual practitioner who requires identification and intervention in order to be restored to health and effective practice.

Furthermore, NNSA believes the nursing profession can meet the above described responsibilities by taking action in the following areas:

Education on the Disease Process of Alcoholism and/or Drug Addiction. Although the American Medical Association and the American Hospital Association designated alcoholism as a disease in 1957, attitudes within the health professions toward persons suffering from chemical dependency have remained largely negative. The person falling victim to it is far too often viewed as weak-willed or morally inferior. Education in nursing schools has been centered around the physical consequences rather than knowledge of how the disease presents itself in the total life of an individual. It is largely a lack of understanding of the psychological defense mechanism of denial that leads to reluctance to intervene when a colleague becomes impaired.

NNSA believes that knowledge of chemical dependency as a disease process should be included in the basic content of every nursing education curriculum. Information in the form of continuing education should be provided to update those nurses educated before such additions to nursing curricula and also to keep all nurses current as the body of knowledge on chemical dependency increases through research and experience.

Furthermore, education specific to the chemically dependent nurse should be provided through in-service education in the various institutions, through workshops providing continuing education credits, and/or through the various state nurses' associations. This education should include practical information regarding recognition of chemical dependency in the nurse as well as the measures to be taken once it is identified.

Employee Assistance Programs. Although industry has demonstrated the cost effectiveness of identifying and treating employees whose job performance has become impaired due to alcoholism and/or drug addiction as well as other emotional problems, institutions employing nurses have generally lagged behind in providing such services to their employees. NNSA believes that all institutions employing nurses should have available a written program that states clearly the policy and procedure in regard to all employees whose job performance has become impaired due to the use of mind-altering drugs. This program should have support from the highest level of management with the institution. Employees should be informed of the program's existence and the mechanism for implementation as part of their orientation. Nursing supervisors should be educated in the technique of documentation of deterioration in job performance and method of confrontation and referral to the employee assistance counselor. The institution should have available as part of its employee assistance program (EAP) a counselor knowledgeable about the nature of chemical dependency and trained in the technique of intervention who can refer for treatment as necessary. Such assistance should be provided before job performance deteriorates to the point that termination is necessary.

Peer Assistance Programs. NNSA takes the position that each of the various states should design and implement a peer assistance program. The threat of loss of licensure can be a powerful tool for penetrating the denial system in which the addicted nurse becomes enmeshed. The design of programs throughout the various states will vary, but certain elements are essential for an effective program.

There should be a mechanism through which calls of concerned persons in reference to an impaired nurse may be received. This can be in the form of a hotline number which is widely publicized. Such a number may be tied in with the impaired physicians' hotline. The caller should be assured confidentiality.

The validity of the concern should be verified to eliminate capricious or vindictive reporting. The method for doing so will be determined by each program.

If the concern appears to be valid, the nurse in question should be called upon by at least two of his or her peers. If possible one of these nurses should be recovering from chemical dependency. These interviewers (or whatever each program chooses to call them) should be knowledgeable about chemical dependency and the techniques of intervention.

The impaired nurse should be offered treatment with some sort of contract, preferably written, in reference to participation in such treatment.

If the nurse refuses to accept treatment, there should be a mechanism for reporting this back to the committee, with some provision for follow-up. Whether the program is designed to have liaison with the State Board of Nursing to report impaired nurses who refuse treatment is up to the individual state.

The attitude of the program should be at all times one of advocacy, not of punishment. Confidentiality of persons involved should be safeguarded.

Nurses Concerned for Nurses. As a mechanism for providing support to nurses recovering from chemical dependency, NNSA supports the concept of nurses across the various states who meet together and are available to reach out to the nurse newly recovering. To this end, NNSA through its Task Force on the Impaired Nurse, is compiling a Directory of Resource Persons who are willing to serve as contact persons. NNSA, through chapters in local areas and as individual members in those areas not yet regionalized, will publicize the existence of this resource. These support groups can give very effective assistance to newly recovering nurses as they face the difficult task of re-entry into practice.

Treatment. NNSA affirms its belief that when a nurse is referred for treatment it should be to a resource trained and knowledgeable in chemical dependency as a primary disease process. Whether such treatment should be as in-patient or out-patient depends on the individual case, the severity of dysfunction, length of addiction, drugs being used, and support system available to the nurse. The goal of treatment for chemical dependency should be total abstinence from all mind-altering drugs except as prescribed by a physician knowledgeable in the field of chemical dependency.

Prepared by the NNSA Task Force on the Impaired Nurse, and adopted by membership March, 1983. Pat Green, RN, MSW, Chairperson, Lawrence, Kansas; Virginia Clarke, RN, Long Beach, California; Jane Meier, RN, CAC, Indianapolis, Indiana; David Roscoe, RN, MEd, Boston, Massachusetts; Liz Karesch, RN, Passiac, New Jersey. Used with permission.

American Association of Nurse Anesthetists
Position Statement on Chemical Dependency

The American Association of Nurse Anesthetists (AANA) expresses its commitment to the promotion of the profession of nurse anesthesia, to the support of all members of the AANA, and to the practice of competent anesthesia care for all consumers. Chemical dependency poses potential threats to these goals, therefore, the AANA recognizes that education, research and resources are the responsibility of the profession in seeking to resolved the issue of chemical dependency.

"Chemically dependent" is defined as the use or abuse of a substance which the person is unable or unwilling to stop the use of, therefore interfering with safe anesthesia practice and personal relationships with family, profession, health and self. The AANA supports the concept of helping nurse anesthetists identified as "chemically dependent" to become "chemically independent."

The AANA affirms that nurse anesthetists are legally and ethically accountable to the consumer and the profession for the quality of anesthesia care rendered.

The AANA recognizes that a safe, supportive and confidential atmosphere is essential to protect the rights of those seeking assistance with chemical dependency.

The AANA has a responsibility to identify and recommend the means of educating anesthesia practitioners to the inherent problems of the chemically dependent, to investigate the availability and effectiveness of treatment modalities, to provide information as to mechanisms of peer support, to recommend research of chemical dependency in nurse anesthesia, and to make recommendation for the provision of care by providing names of available, qualified rehabilitation centers.

Adopted by the AANA Board of Directors 11/84.

Source: American Association of Nurse Anesthetists; Park Ridge, Illinois. Used with permission.

AMERICAN MEDICAL WOMEN'S ASSOCIATION
POSITION STATEMENT ON DRUG TESTING

WHEREAS, Chemical dependency (alcohol and drug abuse) is a serious problem of concern to both medical professionals and the public;

WHEREAS, There is growing concern in this country regarding chemical dependency as an issue of both personal and public health;

WHEREAS, The medical profession recognizes chemical dependency as an illness which responds to treatment;

WHEREAS, Urine screening is being promoted both politically and commercially as a quick and easy solution to this complex problem;

WHEREAS, Indiscriminate drug testing poses serious questions of violation of privacy and due process;

WHEREAS, There is substantial concern regarding the accuracy of drug screening tests, the handling of samples, the quality of laboratory processing, the large numbers of false positives and false negatives;

WHEREAS, Drug screening tests give no information as to the amount or frequency of substance use, or to the degree of impairment;

To encourage rational discussion and protection of individual rights as well as to promote treatment of those afflicted with this illness, be it resolved that: AMWA supports the premise that chemical dependency is a treatable illness and that efforts to identify impaired individuals be within that complex.

And be it resolved that: AMWA supports the development of Federally funded treatment programs and public education programs which utilize well established methods of treatment and intervention, and are available to all individuals chemically dependent and at risk for chemical dependency.

And be it resolved that: AMWA supports the development of programs aimed at addressing chemical dependency and drug testing that include:

The restriction that drug testing be done only as a part of a treatment program and not with punitive consequences and

That there be prohibition of random or mass screening of employees and students and

That there be restriction of testing to those identified as impaired by experts in the treatment of chemical dependency and

That there be mandatory, confirmatory testing on all positive screening tests and

That there be strict guidelines to insure accurate handling of samples and high quality laboratory processing and

That there be treatment of the results of drug screening as part of the medical record and therefore confidential.

Source: American Medical Women's Association; New York., 1986. Used with permission.

APPENDIX E

NATIONAL OFFICES OF MUTUAL HELP OR RESOURCE ORGANIZATIONS

Al-Anon Family Groups, P.O. Box 862, Midtown Station, New York, NY 10018-0862; (212) 302–7240

Alcoholics Anonymous (AA), P.O. Box 459, Grand Central Station, New York, NY 10163; (212) 686–1100.

Anesthetists in Recovery (AIR), c/o Beth Visintine, CRNA, 5626 Preston Oaks Road 40D, Dallas, TX 75240; (214) 960-7296.

Association of Labor-Management Administrators and Consultants to Alcoholism (ALMACA), 1800 North Kent Street, Suite 907, Arlington, VA 22209; (703) 522–6272.

Drug and Alcohol Nursing Association, Inc. (DANA), Carolyn Wittenburg, P.O. Box 6216, Annapolis, MD 21401; (301) 263–1131.

International Advisory Council for Homosexual Men and Women in Alcoholics Anonymous (IAC), P.O. Box 492, Village Station, New York, NY 10014.

National Council on Alcohol, 12 W. 21st Street, New York, NY 10010; (212) 206–6770.

National Institute on Alcohol Abuse and Alcoholism (NIAAA), 5600 Fishers Lane, Rockville, MD 20857.

National Nurses Society on Addictions (NNSA), Impaired Nurse Committee, c/o Pat Green, R.N., 1020 Sunset Drive, Lawrence, KS 66044; (913) 842–3893.

National Self-Help Clearinghouse (NSHC), City University of New York, 33 West 42nd Street, New York, NY 10036. (Letters only, please.)

Women for Sobriety, Inc., P.O. Box 618, Quakertown, PA 18951; (215) 536–8026.

NATIONAL NURSES SOCIETY ON ADDICTIONS' STATEMENT ON MODEL DIVERSION LEGISLATION FOR CHEMICALLY DEPENDENT NURSES

Over recent years, state nurses associations, specialty nursing groups and others, have worked to develop positions, mechanisms and peer assistance programs to help impaired nurses. Their goal(s) have been to assist nurses, whose practice is either actually or potentially affected, to find appropriate treatment for their illness, thus assisting and protecting both nurse and patient.

The nurse suffering from the primary illness of alcohol and/or drug addiction has long been a concern, not just of the profession, but also state regulatory bodies. State nursing boards have as their primary function, the protection of the public. In fulfilling that responsibility, they have often been in the position of being required to discipline a nurse for an act of commission or omission resulting purely from what is acknowledged to be the nurse's illness. Few boards have been pleased with this requirement, but have not felt that alternatives were available to them.

The National Nurses Society on Addictions, after observing the legislative efforts of such states as Florida, California and Hawaii, the programs developed by other professions, and the handling of other violations requiring due process, believes that a model diversion program for nurses, to be adopted by each state, could be of great assistance to the Boards of Nursing, individual nurses, our profession and our patients.

The following is a model statement and diversion legislation that NNSA hopes will be helpful in dealing with this issue in a safe, effective and humane manner.

Model Statement

The _____ State Board of Nursing, in the matter of nurses whose functioning is impaired by alcoholism or drug addiction, recognizes:

1. that alcoholism and drug addiction are primary illnesses and should be treated as such.

2. that problems resulting from these illnesses can include personal, legal and health problems that may impair the nurse's personal health and ability to practice safely.

3. that nurses who develop these illnesses can, with appropriate treatment, be helped to recover.

4. that programs of assistance that include treatment and monitoring, as an alternative to a disciplinary process, have been particularly effective in rehabilitating the professional and in protecting the public.

5. that nurses who are willing to cooperate with a program of assistance to them and accept treatment for these illness should be allowed to avoid disciplinary action provided they cooperate fully with recommended treatment and comply with the requirements for monitoring of their continued well-being after formal treatment is completed.

Therefore, the _____ State Board of Nursing supports the enactment of an amendment to the nurse practice act in this state calling for a diversion procedure for nurses who have been (or are likely to be) charged with violating the nurse practice act, but who are willing to stipulate to certain facts and enter a program approved by the Board.

Diversion Procedure

Section _____ .

It is the intent of the Legislature that the Board of Nursing (hereinafter referred to as the Board) seek ways and means to identify and rehabilitate nurses whose competency may be impaired due to abuse of drugs or alcohol, so that such nurses can be treated and can return to or continue the practice of nursing in a manner which will benefit the public. It is further the intent of the Legislature that the Board of Nursing, by implementing this legislation, will establish a diversion procedure as a voluntary alternative to traditional disciplinary actions and as an alternative to lengthy and costly investigations and administrative proceedings against such nurses but also having adequate safeguards for the patient.

Section _____ .

As used in this statute:

1. "Program" means a formal, structured regimen, sponsored by a recognized group, designed to and capable of assisting addicted nurses and referring them for evaluation and treatment, including mutual help groups and monitoring them for a period of at least two years.

   a.   "Peer Assistance Program" means a program administered by professional nurses for the purpose of assisting their colleagues in obtaining evaluation, treatment, monitoring and on-going support for the purpose of arresting their addiction.

   b.   "Employee Assistance Program" means a program offered by an employer of nurses for the purpose of identifying and assisting them in obtaining evaluation, treatment, monitoring and on-going support for the purpose of arresting their addiction.

   c.   "Approved Program" means either a Peer Assistance Program or an Employee Assistance Program that has been approved and accepted by the Board of Nursing as having the ability to meet the requirements of this act by referring nurses for evaluation and treatment and by providing on-going support and monitoring for those nurses.

2. "Treatment" refers to a formalized plan carried out by a chemical dependency professional in either an in-patient or out-patient setting, designed to provide primary care, leading to rehabilitation.

3. "Committee" refers to a Diversion Evaluation Committee appointed by the Board to carry out such duties as are herein described.

Section _____ .

The Board shall appoint one or more Diversion Evaluation Committees.

1. The Committee will be composed of five persons:

   a.   two registered nurses and once licensed practical nurse, all licensed under this chapter. The Board will give consideration to recommendations of nursing organizations and shall give priority consideration to the appointment of nurses who have recovered from impairment or who specialize in addictions nursing.

b.   two members not necessarily licensed as nurses but who have experience or knowledge in the evaluation or management of persons impaired by chemical dependency.

2. Each appointment shall be at the pleasure of the Board for a term not to exceed four years. The Board, at its discretion, may stagger the terms of the initial members appointed. A member may be reappointed once.

3. The members of the Committee will serve without pay, but will be reimbursed for the expenses incurred in the discharge of their duties at a rate determined by the state for all state business.

4. The Committee shall elect a chairperson and a vice-chairperson.

5. The Committee will review the request of each nurse for diversion, according to criteria established by the Board, and recommend to the Board either in favor or against diversion. In all cases where the Committee has recommended diversion the Board shall grant diversion, except that for good cause shown the Board may disregard the Committee's recommendation and deny diversion.

6. The Committee will review the regimen developed by a Program for each nurse and will determine whether that nurse may safely continue or resume the practice of nursing while on diversion.

7. The Committee will hear reports from the nurses on diversion and from the Program as to each nurse's progress and cooperation and will, in turn, report and refer to the Board all relevant information and requests for action according to guidelines established by the Board.

Section _____ .

One or more programs may be designated and contracted with as approved programs by the Board to carry out this article. Such programs must meet the following requirements:

1. Peer Assistance Programs will be designated for approval by the Board after consideration of the recommendation of the Committee and providing:

    a.   they are sponsored by or in conjunction with the state nurses' association.

    b.   that staff and/or volunteers of the program are educated, experienced, and supervised, appropriate to the level of involvement in the program.

c.   they include within their program, referral to bona fide chemical dependency treatment centers, e.g., those accredited by the Joint Commission on the Accreditation of Hospitals or those licensed by the state as such.

d.   they refer to mutual help groups, e.g., Alcoholics Anonymous, Narcotics Anonymous.

e.   they monitor participants for a period of two years including the random examination of body fluids as appropriate.

f.   they agree to immediately report to the Committee, any nurse that does not cooperate and comply with the requirements of the program.

g.   they agree to report to the Committee, regularly and when requested, the status of individual nurses as to cooperation and progress, including the overall status of the Program.

2. Employee Assistance Programs will be designated Programs for approval by the Board after consideration of the recommendation of the Committee providing:

a.   they have staff that have had a minimum of two years experience in the addictions field and in a health care agency or are directly supervised by someone with such experience.

b.   they include within their programs, referral to bona fide chemical dependency treatment centers, e.g., those accredited by the Joint Commission on the Accreditation of Hospitals or those licensed by the state as such.

c.   they refer to mutual help groups, e.g., Alcoholics Anonymous, Narcotics Anonymous.

d.   they monitor participants for a period of two years including the use of random drug screens.

e.   they agree to immediately report to the Committee, any nurse that does not cooperate and comply with the requirements of the program.

f.   they agree to report to the Committee, regularly and when requested, the status of individual nurses as to cooperation and progress and the overall status of the Program.

If no suitable programs are available in the state, the Board may contract for the development of such a program, providing it has no direct control over the program.

Section _____ .

The Board may increase the licensing fee for each nurse in the state, not to exceed $5, to cover the cost of implementation and maintenance of this article.

Section _____ .

Any nurse appearing before the Board for a violation of the nurse practice act due to an apparent addiction to alcohol or other drugs will be advised of the opportunity for diversion. The nurse will be advised of the procedure to be followed and to be eligible, such nurse must stipulate to certain facts, waive a speedy hearing or trial and become a participant in, and agree to cooperate with, an approved program. The Board may grant diversion to a nurse after reviewing the nurse's application for diversion and the recommendation of the Committee. Subsequent failure to cooperate and comply shall be reported to the Board by the Committee and may result in termination of the diversion procedure.

Section _____ .

The Board of Nursing will develop a written diversion agreement which sets forth the requirements which must be met by the nurse and the conditions under which the diversion procedure may be successfully completed or terminated due to lack of cooperation or compliance. Time already spent in an approved program may be taken into consideration by the Board in determining the length of diversion.

Section _____ .

Records of the approved programs and treatment as they pertain to the diversion procedure shall be kept confidential, with the exception of the reporting as to whether or not the nurse is cooperating and complying, and are not subject to discovery or subpoena.

Section _____ .

During the time the nurse is on diversion he or she will be required to remain in an approved program. Participation in a satisfactory program in another state may be approved upon application and a showing of need. The diversionee may not practice in another state without the knowledge of the Board of that state of his/her participation in the diversion procedure.

Section _____ .

After a period of five years, provided no additional occurrences of alcohol or drug related violations or crimes have occurred, the records of the diversion and charges will be purged upon request of the nurse.

Section _____ .

Any person making reports to the Board or to the Committee regarding a nurse suspected of practicing while impaired or reports of a nurse's progress or lack of progress in a Program shall be immune from civil action for defamation or other cause of action resulting from such reports, provided that such report is made in good faith and with some reasonable basis in fact.

Section _____ .

The Board of Nursing, any Committee or member thereof appointed by the Board, any Program or its staff or volunteers, any Treatment agency or its staff or volunteers, or any nurse, licensed to practice under the laws of this State that has supervisor responsibility over the practice of nursing by a diversionee, or an employer of such a diversionee, shall not be liable for any civil damages resulting from the diversionee's negligence in his/her practice, or the fact that such diversionee's license to practice was not revoked, or that such diversionee was employed or retained in employment except for such damages which may result from such person, Board or group's negligence or wanton acts or omissions in the supervision of the impaired nurse.

Caution

Mandatory reporting is not included in this model. This is a difficult issue and is felt to be, in general, counter-productive. Should it be in force in certain states or considered for inclusion with this proposed legislation, an exemption should be allowed for those nurses working in treatment programs or programs of assistance.

We suggest that close attention be paid to the section on the funding of the act. It should be clear that the Board can use that money to pay for the cost of programs when needed.

Persons not familiar with the legislative process should be warned that the passage of the act is not the final action. The drafting of the rules and regulations and guidelines that implement the act are also important and will require the attention of interested persons.

Source: National Nurses Society on Addictions; Evanston, IL. Used with permission.

Employee Assistance Program (EAP) Model

By Etta Williams, MPA, RN, SCADC

Note: An effective EAP is one that addresses all employees, professional and supportive. It should identify troubled employees early, *before* serious problems occur and offer monitoring for an extended period when the employee returns to the work setting, *after it is determined that he or she is capable of resuming their duties.* EAPs can be as extensive as the needs of the organization demand, but they can also be very simple and can easily be implemented by a hospital or agency of any size. The following are suggested policies and procedures. It would be necessary to adapt them to a particular situation.

Purpose

The purpose of the Employee Assistance Program at _____
Hospital is to promote safe patient care and the health and well being of the employees of this hospital. The confidentiality of the employees utilizing this program will be respected and protected except when to do so could endanger a patient, the employee, or someone else.

POLICY

Since all persons in our society, including the employees of _____
Hospital, are susceptible to illness that may impair their ability to function
at an optimal level, and since these illnesses, including chemical
dependency, are frequently illnesses that can be successfully treated, it is
the policy of this hospital to treat employees having such illnesses as
employees with other illnesses are treated in respect to their retention,
performance, and the use of sick leave and other benefits. These benefits are
available to employees that are self referred and to those referred by their
supervisors, who have identified a performance problem and are utilizing
this program as an adjunct to the normal disciplinary process. Available
sick time will be used for the evaluation and any treatment required. The
EAP program may be offered to an employee by a supervisor at any point in
the disciplinary process and always before termination, providing the
employee agrees to be evaluated by an approved treatment program and to
sign a release allowing that program to communicate freely with the EAP
coordinator.

   If found to be chemically dependent, or to have any other illness or
condition that has the potential to impair judgement and/or performance,
the employee agrees to:

1. enter into and continue with treatment as recommended.

2. close supervision of professional practice and an understanding that
    satisfactory job performance must be maintained.

   If the employee is diagnosed as having chemical dependency or any
other illness or condition that involves the potential for the diversion or
mishandling of drugs, including alcohol and medication, the employee
further agrees to:

3. not use any mood altering drug of addiction (all medications that might
    be prescribed must be approved by the EAP coordinator and the
    therapist and consultation with a physician knowledgeable in chemical
    dependency may be required) and to cooperate with body fluid drug
    screens as requested to monitor this requirement.

4. participate in an approved peer assistance program if one is available to
    them for a period of not less than two years.

5. not administer or otherwise handle any mood altering chemicals until
    certain conditions are met and a recommendation is made by the
    therapist and/or peer assistance monitor and approved by the supervisor.

6. participate in a mutual help group on a continued basis at not less than two meetings per week unless otherwise recommended by their therapist.

7. sign an agreement including the above conditions as they apply and specifying that if those conditions are not met, that the licensing board (if applicable) will be notified and they will be terminated.

Implementation

The Employee Assistance Program of _____ Hospital will be implemented as follows:

The EAP coordinator will be named

The policy as articulated herein will be distributed to all employees and their families

Educational programs will be offered on the subjects of:

a.   illnesses that can result in impaired performance, including signs, symptoms and characteristics

b.   laws, rules and regulations pertaining to impaired practice

c.   the policies of this hospital including identification, reporting and return to work requirements.

Related Policies

To be added to the Fitness for Duty Policy:
If an employee is taking a drug that has been prescribed by a physician, but could impair the employee's ability to practice safely, the employee must notify the supervisor and the employee health nurse and sign a release of information for the hospital designee to talk with the physician. The supervisor, the employee health nurse and the hospital risk manager will determine whether or not the employee may continue to work or be placed on sick leave.

Alcohol use or the use of other drugs or medications that have the potential to impair judgement and/or motor skills, immediately preceding or during the hours of work is not acceptable. All employees have the obligation to report such use by other employees, or anyone delivering service in this hospital, to their supervisor or the risk manager.

An employee may observe other actions or behaviors in a co-worker that could indicate a person is unable to perform safely and these should be reported to a supervisor immediately. Examples (not all inclusive) are:

- bizarre or inappropriate behavior
- unexplained, unusual or excessive numbers of medication errors
- errors in judgement in patient care
- frequent disappearances from the work site
- possible drug diversion

In the event an employee is suspected of using alcohol or other drugs or of diverting drugs intended for a patient to their own use, regardless of the drug involved, this suspicion will be reported to the employee's supervisor immediately, who is then required to report and consult with the hospital's risk manager. An investigation will be conducted to determine the possible validity of the report. If the investigation reveals that impaired practice exists, or is likely to exist, the supervisor must consult with the person(s) named above and immediate steps to protect the patients will be implemented. Careful, complete and confidential documentation must be maintained of all steps taken.

Persons involved in making such reports or the investigation of reports should avoid discussing the report or its contents with other hospital personnel.

Should a supervisor have reason to believe an employee has used alcohol or other drugs or diverted drugs, either by their own observations or the report of another person, the employee will be asked to submit to a body fluid examination and will be relieved of duty. Disciplinary steps to be taken will be determined after the results of such tests are available, but will depend on the behavior involved as well as the results of the tests. Should the tests be negative and no behavior has occurred that would warrant disciplinary action, the employee will receive full pay for the time off and all records of the incident will be removed from their files.

To Be Added to the Policy on Health Care Benefits:
Since it is the policy of this hospital's health benefits program to provide coverage to treat all illnesses that may occur in the employee group, as of this date, mental illness, alcoholism and other drug addictions will be covered by the health plan.

To Be Added to the Policy on Work Performance:
Satisfactory work performance is required in order to retain employment in this hospital. Unsatisfactory work performance that is possibly the result of an illness still requires the implementation of the counseling/disciplinary procedure on the part of the supervisor. The supervisor may be made aware of actual or potential impaired work performance by:

- their own direct observations

- reporting systems or summaries of reports indicating trends that could affect job performance

- reports from other staff, written or verbal

- reports from patients

Once made aware of the problem, the supervisor must investigate and consult with the risk manager (see policy on Fitness-for-Duty).

Model Agreement When an Employee Is Referred to the EAP by a Supervisor

_____ Hospital Employee Assistance Program Agreement

I, _____ , an employee of _____ Hospital, understand that there are legitimate concerns about my performance and in an attempt to improve that performance to an acceptable level, I agree to be evaluated, using my sick leave as necessary, by an approved treatment program and to sign a release of information allowing that program to communicate with the EAP coordinator of this hospital and if found to be chemically dependent, or to have any other illness or condition that has the potential to impair judgement and/or performance, I agree to:

1. enter into and continue with treatment as recommended, using my sick leave as it is available.

2. close supervision of my performance and I understand that a satisfactory job performance must be maintained.

If I am diagnosed as chemically dependent or am determined to have any other illness or condition that involves the potential for the diversion or mishandling of drugs including alcohol and medications, I additionally agree to:

3. not use any mood altering drug of addiction (all medications that might be prescribed must be approved by my therapist and the EAP coordinator and consultation with a physician knowledgeable in chemical dependency may be required) and to cooperate with body fluid drug screens as requested to monitor this requirement.

4. participate in an approved peer assistance program if one is available to me for a period of not less than two years.

5. not administer or otherwise handle any mood altering chemicals until certain conditions are met and a recommendation is made by my therapist and/or peer assistance monitor and approved by my supervisor.

6. participate in a mutual help group on a continued basis at no less than two meetings per week unless otherwise recommended by my therapist.

7. and understand that if these conditions are not met, the Board of _____ Hospital will be notified and I will be terminated immediately.

Signed: _____ Date:_____
Witnessed: _____

APPENDIX H

State Board of Nursing Licensure Violations and Actions—1985

1985 State Board–Reported Violations Involving Drugs/Alcohol

STATE	NUMBER OF NURSES	TOTAL CASES	CASES PER 1000 NURSES	DRUG/ALCOHOL CASES	% RELATED TO DRUG/ALCOHOL
California	237,358	172	.7	125	73
Pennsylvania	177,152	83	.4	34	41
Texas	159,435	293	1.8	190	65
Ohio	135,064	21	.1	15	71
Illinois	130,538	65	.5	57	88
Florida	120,503	239	1.9	132	55
Michigan	107,239	48	.4	42	88
Massachusetts	105,898	98	.9	98	100
New Jersey	95,049	60	.6	55	92
Georgia (RN only)	36,304	44	.7	34	77
North Carolina	58,503	66	1.1	47	71
Virginia	58,156	93	1.6	77	83
Minnesota	56,745	66	1.1	25	38

STATE	NUMBER OF NURSES	TOTAL CASES	CASES PER 1000 NURSES	DRUG/ALCOHOL CASES	% RELATED TO DRUG/ALCOHOL
Wisconsin	54,725	38	.7	28	74
Indiana	53,197	9	.1	7	78
Tennessee	48,361	42	.8	35	83
Connecticut	45,810	28	.6	19	68
Alabama	41,221	75	1.0	63	84
Iowa	39,403	39	1.0	10	26
Colorado	38,187	68	1.7	50	74
Louisiana	37,203	116	3.1	101	87
Kentucky	28,431	91	3.2	28	31
Oregon	27,986	109	4.0	39	36
South Carolina	27,249	61	2.2	57	93
Mississippi	23,562	58	2.5	43	74
West Virginia	19,699	14	.7	9	64
New Hampshire	14,877	15	1.0	12	80
Rhode Island	14,298	16	1.1	12	75
New Mexico	12,560	22	1.8	15	68
Utah	12,395	25	2.0	17	68
Hawaii	11,108	4	.3	4	100
Montana	9,943	10	1.0	7	70
Idaho	9,834	21	2.3	13	62
North Dakota	9,655	9	.9	5	56
Vermont	7,994	9	1.2	7	78
Nevada	7,663	13	1.8	4	31
Wyoming	4,272	15	3.7	4	27
Total	2,100,105	2,255	50.5	1,520	67

Source: Anita Chesney, North Carolina Board of Nursing. Used with permission.

1985 State Board Disciplinary Actions in Alcohol and Drug Related Cases

STATE	NUMBER OF ALCOHOL/ DRUG CASES	NUMBER OF DISCIPLINARY ACTIONS*	ACTIONS TAKEN									
			REPRIMANDS		PROBATIONS		SUSPENSIONS		REVOCATIONS		OTHER RESTRICTIONS	
			No.	(%)	No.	(%)	No.	(%)	No.	(%)	No.	(%)
Texas	190	217	6	(3)	33	(15)	73	(34)	59	(27)	46	(21)
Florida	132	132	6	(5)	54	(41)	43	(32)	11	(8)	18	(14)
California	125	162	0	(0)	91	(56)	3	(2)	65	(40)	3	(2)
Louisiana	101	111	1	(1)	40	(36)	37	(33)	13	(12)	20	(18)
Massachusetts	98	98	36	(37)	30	(31)	1	(1)	0	(0)	31	(32)
Virginia	77	77	2	(3)	38	(49)	33	(43)	4	(5)	0	(0)
Alabama	63	63	0	(0)	27	(43)	1	(2)	7	(11)	28	(44)
Illinois	57	57	0	(0)	26	(46)	25	(44)	6	(11)	0	(0)
South Carolina	57	57	0	(0)	0	(0)	21	(37)	3	(5)	33	(58)
New Jersey	55	88	2	(3)	25	(28)	23	(26)	12	(14)	26	(29)
Colorado	50	45	4	(9)	5	(11)	5	(11)	6	(13)	25	(56)
North Carolina	47	47	3	(6)	0	(0)	10	(21)	11	(23)	23	(49)
Mississippi	43	37	0	(0)	6	(16)	0	(0)	25	(68)	6	(16)
Michigan	42	42	3	(7)	4	(10)	24	(57)	9	(21)	2	(5)
Oregon	39	39	0	(0)	9	(23)	22	(56)	4	(10)	4	(10)
Tennessee	35	35	0	(0)	10	(28)	7	(20)	16	(46)	2	(6)
Pennsylvania	34	79	22	(28)	24	(30)	1	(1)	7	(9)	25	(32)
Georgia (RNs only)	34	34	0	(0)	0	(0)	1	(3)	0	(0)	33	(97)
Kentucky	28	28	0	(0)	4	(14)	10	(36)	0	(0)	14	(50)
Wisconsin	28	28	0	(0)	0	(0)	2	(8)	8	(29)	18	(64)
Minnesota	25	25	0	(0)	0	(0)	16	(64)	3	(12)	6	(24)

STATE	NUMBER OF ALCOHOL/ DRUG CASES	NUMBER OF DISCIPLINARY ACTIONS*	ACTIONS TAKEN									
			REPRIMANDS		PROBATIONS		SUSPENSIONS		REVOCATIONS		OTHER RESTRICTIONS	
			No.	(%)	No.	(%)	No.	(%)	No.	(%)	No.	(%)
Connecticut	19	19	0	(0)	1	(5)	12	(63)	1	(5)	5	(26)
Utah	17	17	0	(0)	7	(41)	3	(18)	4	(24)	3	(18)
New Mexico	15	15	0	(0)	3	(20)	3	(20)	3	(20)	6	(40)
Ohio	15	15	0	(0)	0	(0)	4	(27)	9	(60)	2	(13)
Idaho	13	13	2	(15)	0	(0)	2	(15)	2	(15)	7	(54)
Rhode Island	12	16	2	(13)	1	(6)	3	(19)	0	(0)	10	(63)
New Hampshire	12	13	1	(8)	4	(31)	5	(38)	1	(8)	2	(15)
Iowa	10	10	0	(0)	7	(70)	1	(10)	1	(10)	1	(10)
West Virginia	9	13	0	(0)	4	(31)	5	(38)	0	(0)	4	(31)
Montana	7	7	0	(0)	4	(57)	3	(43)	0	(0)	0	(0)
Vermont	7	7	0	(0)	1	(14)	6	(86)	0	(0)	0	(0)
Indiana	7	7	0	(0)	2	(29)	3	(43)	2	(29)	0	(0)
North Dakota	5	5	0	(0)	1	(20)	0	(0)	1	(20)	3	(60)
Wyoming	4	4	0	(0)	1	(25)	0	(0)	2	(50)	1	(25)
Nevada	4	4	0	(0)	1	(25)	0	(0)	3	(75)	0	(0)
Hawaii	4	4	0	(0)	0	(0)	3	(75)	0	(0)	1	(25)
Total	1520	1670	90	(5)	463	(28)	411	(25)	298	(18)	408	(24)

*The number of disciplinary actions may be greater than the number of cases due to multiple actions relating to one case.

Source: Anita Chesney, North Carolina Board of Nursing. Used with permission.

APPENDIX I

AMERICAN NURSES' ASSOCIATION CODE FOR NURSES

PREAMBLE

The Code for Nurses is based on belief about the nature of individuals, nursing, health, and society. Recipients and providers of nursing services are viewed as individuals and groups who possess basic rights and responsibilities, and whose values and circumstances command respect at all times. Nursing encompasses the promotion and restoration of health, the prevention of illness, and the alleviation of suffering. The statements of the Code and their interpretation provide guidance for conduct and relationships in carrying out nursing responsibilities consistent with the ethical obligations of the profession and quality in nursing care.

CODE FOR NURSES

1. The nurse provides services with respect for human dignity and the uniqueness of the client, unrestricted by considerations of social or economic status, personal attributes, or the nature of health problems.

2. The nurse safeguards the client's right to privacy by judiciously protecting information of a confidential nature.

3. The nurse acts to safeguard the client and the public when health care and safety are affected by the incompetent, unethical, or illegal practice of any person.

4. The nurse assumes responsibility and accountability for individual nursing judgments and actions.

5. The nurse maintains competence in nursing.

6. The nurse exercises informed judgment and uses individual competence and qualifications as criteria in seeking consultation, accepting responsibilities, and delegating nursing activities to others.

7. The nurse participates in activities that contribute to the ongoing development of the profession's body of knowledge.

8. The nurse participates in the profession's efforts to implement and improve standards of nursing.

9. The nurse participates in the profession's efforts to establish and maintain conditions of employment conducive to high quality nursing care.

10. The nurse participates in the profession's effort to protect the public from misinformation and misrepresentation and to maintain the integrity of nursing.

11. The nurse collaborates with members of the health professions and other citizens in promoting community and national efforts to meet the health needs of the public.

Source: American Nurses' Association, Inc. Used with permission. (For a complete statement of standards with interpretive statements, write the Publications Fulfillment Center, 2420 Pershing Road, Kansas City, Missouri 64108.)

APPENDIX J

SCREENING TESTS FOR CHEMICAL DEPENDENCY

MICHIGAN ALCOHOLISM SCREENING TEST (MAST)

POINTS			YES	NO
	0.	Do you enjoy a drink now and then?	___	___
(2)	*1.	Do you feel you are a normal drinker? (By normal we mean you drink less or as much as most other people.)	___	___
(2)	2.	Have you ever awakened the morning after doing some drinking the night before and found that you could not remember a part of the evening?	___	___
(1)	3.	Does your wife, husband, a parent, or other near relative ever worry or complain about your drinking?	___	___
(2)	*4.	Can you stop drinking without a struggle after one or two drinks?	___	___
(1)	5.	Do you ever feel guilty about your drinking?	___	___

---

* Alcoholic response is negative.

POINTS   YES   NO

(2)   *6.   Do friends or relatives think you are a normal drinker?

                                                                ___   ___

(2)   *7.   Are you able to stop drinking when you want to?

                                                                ___   ___

(5)   8.   Have you ever attended a meeting of Alcoholics Anonymous
             (AA)?   ___   ___

(1)   9.   Have you gotten into physical fights when drinking?

                                                                ___   ___

(2)   10.   Has your drinking ever created problems between you and
             your wife, husband, a parent, or other relative?   ___   ___

(2)   11.   Has your wife, husband (or other family members) ever gone
             to anyone for help about your drinking?   ___   ___

(2)   12.   Have you ever lost friends because of your drinking?

                                                                ___   ___

(2)   13.   Have you ever gotten into trouble at work or school because
             of drinking?   ___   ___

(2)   14.   Have you ever lost a job because of drinking?   ___   ___

(2)   15.   Have you ever neglected your obligations, your family, or your
             work for two or more days in a row because you were drinking?

                                                                ___   ___

(1)   16.   Do you drink before noon fairly often?   ___   ___

(2)   17.   Have you ever been told you have liver trouble? Cirrhosis?

                                                                ___   ___

(2)   **18. After heavy drinking have you ever had Delirium Tremens
             (D.T.'s) or severe shaking, or heard voices or seen things that
             really weren't there?   ___   ___

(5)   19.   Have you ever gone to anyone for help about your drinking?

                                                                ___   ___

(5)   20.   Have you ever been in a hospital because of drinking?

                                                                ___   ___

---

* Alcoholic response is negative.

** 5 points for Delirium Tremens

POINTS   YES   NO

(2) 21. Have you ever been a patient in a psychiatric hospital or on a
          psychiatric ward of a general hospital where drinking was part
          of the problem that resulted in hospitalization?   ____   ____

(2) 22. Have you ever been seen at a psychiatric or mental health clinic
          or gone to any doctor, social worker, or clergyman for help with
          any emotional problem, where drinking was part of the problem?

                                                                    ____   ____

(2) ***23. Have you ever been arrested for drunk driving, driving while
          intoxicated, or drinking under the influence of alcoholic
          beverages?   ____   ____

          (If YES, how many times? _____)

(2) ***24. Have you ever been arrested, or taken into custody, even for a
          few hours, because of other drunk behavior?   ____   ____

          (If YES, how many times? _____)

*** 2 points for *each* arrest

Scoring System: In general, five points or more would place the subject in
an "alcoholic" category. Four points would be suggestive of alcoholism,
three points or less would indicate the subject was not alcoholic.

Programs using the above scoring system find it very sensitive at the five
point level and it tends to find more people alcoholic than anticipated.
However, it is a screening test and should be sensitive at its lower levels.

Source: Selzer, M.L. (1971). The Michigan Alcoholism Screening Test (MAST): The
Quest for a New Diagnostic Instrument. *American Journal of Psychiatry*, 3:176–181.
Used with permission.

SHORT MICHIGAN ALCOHOLISM SCREENING TEST (SMAST)

1. Do you feel you are a normal drinker? (By normal we mean you drink less than or as much as most other people.) (No)*

2. Does your wife, husband, a parent, or other near relative ever worry or complain about your drinking? (Yes)

3. Do you ever feel guilty about your drinking? (Yes)

4. Do friends or relatives think you are a normal drinker? (No)

5. Are you able to stop drinking when you want to? (No)

6. Have you ever attended a meeting of Alcoholics Anonymous? (Yes)

7. Has drinking ever created problems between you and your wife, husband, a parent, or other near relative? (Yes)

8. Have you ever gotten into trouble at work because of drinking? (Yes)

9. Have you ever neglected your obligations, your family, or your work for two or more days in a row because you were drinking? (Yes)

10. Have you ever gone to anyone for help about your drinking? (Yes)

11. Have you ever been in a hospital because of drinking? (Yes)

12. Have you ever been arrested for drunken driving, driving while intoxicated, or driving under the influence of alcoholic beverages? (Yes)

13. Have you ever been arrested, even for a few hours, because of other drunken behavior? (Yes)

Source: Selzer, M.L., Vinokur, A,. Evon Rooijen, L. (1975). A self-administered short Michigan Alcoholism Screening Test (SMAST). *Journal of Studies on Alcohol*, 36(1), 117–126. Used with permission.

*Alcoholism-indicating responses in parentheses.

ALCOHOLISM SCREENING TEXT (CAGE)

1. Have you ever felt you ought to Cut down on your drinking?

2. Have people Annoyed you by criticizing your drinking?

3. Have you ever felt bad or Guilty about your drinking?

4. Have you ever had a drink first thing in the morning to steady your nerves or get rid of a hangover (Eye-opener)?

Source: Ewing, J.A. (1984). Detecting alcoholism: The CAGE questionnaire. *JAMA*, 252(14), 1905–1906. Used with permission.

Drug Abuse Screening Test (DAST)

1. Have you used drugs other than those required for medical reasons?

2. Have you abused prescription drugs?

3. Do you abuse more than one drug at a time?

*4. Can you get through the week without using drugs (other than those required for medical reasons)?

*5. Are you always able to stop using drugs when you want to?

6. Do you abuse drugs on a continuous basis?

*7. Do you try to limit your drug use to certain situations?

8. Have you had "blackouts" or "flashbacks" as a result of drug use?

9. Do you ever feel bad about your drug use?

10. Does your spouse (or parents) ever complain about your involvement with drugs?

11. Do your friends or relatives know or suspect you abuse drugs?

12. Has drug abuse ever created problems between you and your spouse?

13. Has any family member ever sought help for problems related to your drug use?

14. Have you ever lost friends because of your use of drugs?

15. Have you ever neglected your family or missed work because of your use of drugs?

16. Have you ever been in trouble at work because of drug use?

17. Have you ever lost a job because of drug abuse?

18. Have you gotten into fights when under the influence of drugs?

19. Have you ever been arrested because of unusual behavior while under the influence of drugs?

20. Have you ever been arrested while driving while under the influence of drugs?

21. Have you engaged in illegal activities in order to obtain drugs?

22. Have you ever been arrested for possession of illegal drugs?

---

*Items 4, 5, and 7 are scored in the "no" or false direction.

23. Have you ever experienced withdrawal symptoms as a result of heavy drug intake?

24. Have you had medical problems as a result of your drug use (eg, memory loss, hepatitis, convulsions, bleeding, etc.)?

25. Have you ever gone to anyone for help for a drug problem?

26. Have you ever been in a hospital for medical problems related to your drug use?

27. Have you ever been involved in a treatment program specifically related to drug use?

28. Have you been treated as an outpatient for problems related to drug abuse?

INDEX

A

AA. *See* Alcoholics Anonymous
Abstinence, monitoring for, 78–84
Addiction. *See* Chemical dependency
Adult Children of Alcoholics, 63
AIDS, 54, 62
Al-Anon, 4, 29, 61–63, 90, 127, 157
Alcohol, 3, 4. *See* also Alcoholism; Drinking
    age and, 15
    benzodiazepines and, 71
    chemically dependent nurse and 27–28
    cocaine user and, 5
    dependency, 4
        disulfiram and, 67–68
        nurses and, 15
        nursing education and, 120–121
    depressive effects of, 6
    diabetes and, 121
    disulfiram reaction with, 68
    excretion rate and, 104
    grand mal seizures and, 121

Continued

Continued

H
Heroin
　　detection period for, 104
　　methadone substitution for, 69
Hospital drugs, chemically dependent nurse and, 26–27
Hypertension, alcohol and, 121
Hypnotics
　　long-term effects of, 50
　　withdrawal, 57

I
Individual therapy, chemical dependency treatment and, 60–61
Insomnia, alcohol withdrawal and, 122
International Advisory Council for Homosexual Men and Women in
　　AA, 157
Intervention, 34–48
　　combined approaches in, 44–46
　　employment-related, 43
　　Johnsonian, 41
　　peer, 41–42
　　planning, 46–48

J
Johnson Institute, 41
Johnsonian intervention, 41
Joint Commission on the Accreditation of Hospitals, 66, 128
Judgment, drinking and, 5

L
Librium. *See* Chlordiazepoxide
Licensure disciplinary actions, state board-reported, 171–172
Licensure sanctions, chemically dependent nurse and, 16–17
Licensure violations, state board-reported, 171–172
Lithium, chemical dependency treatment and, 72

M
Make Today Count, 62
Marijuana, 4, 27
　　addiction, gender and, 12
　　age and, 15
　　detection period for, 104
MAST. *See* Michigan Alcoholism Screening Text